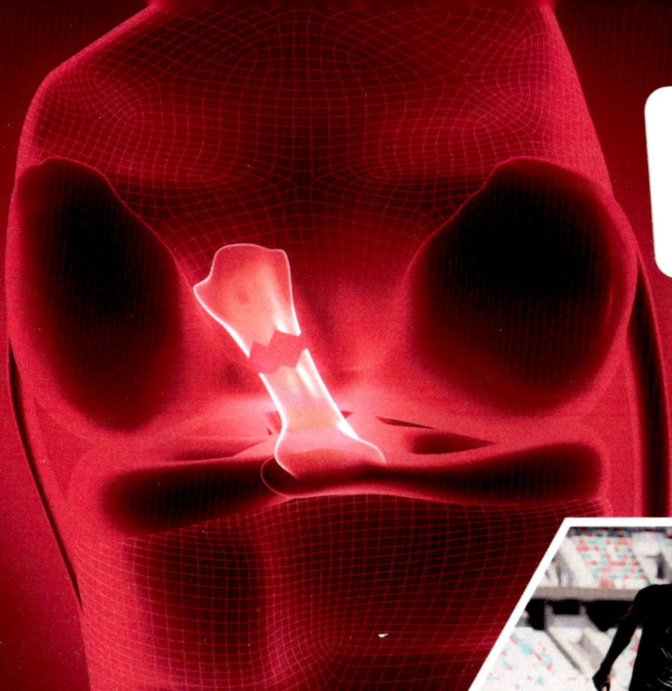

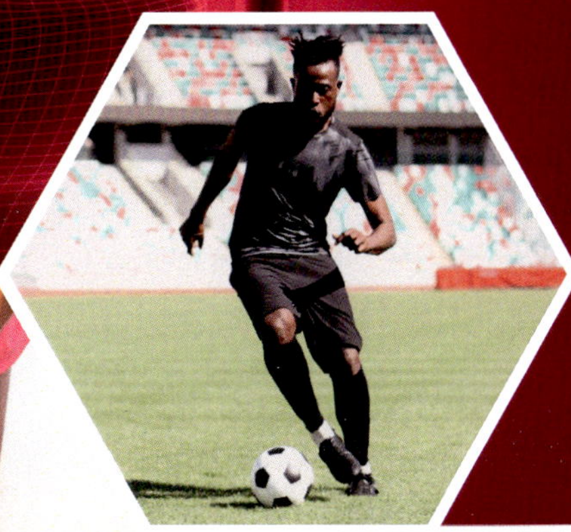

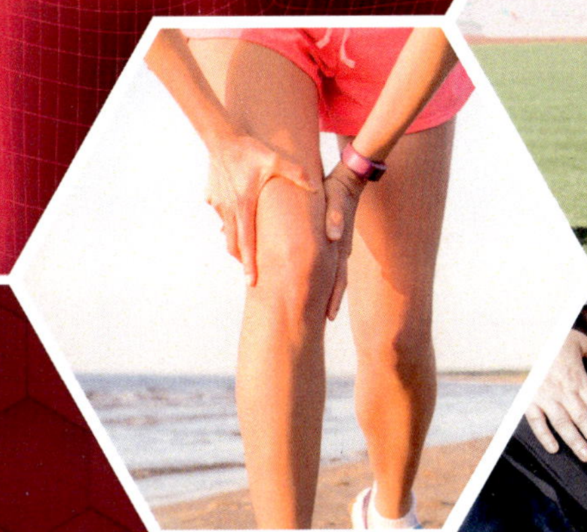

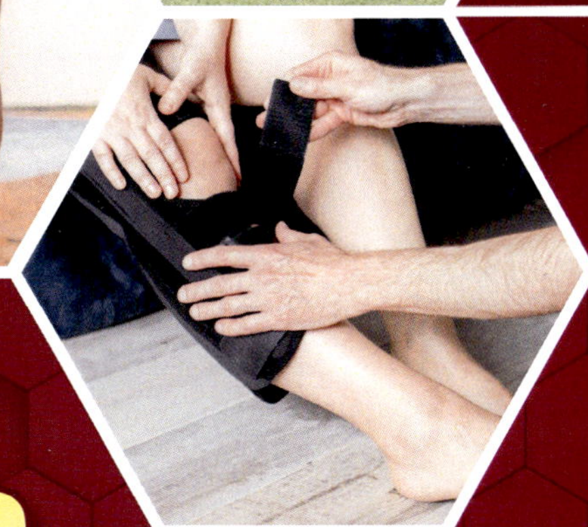

India James

SPORTS INJURIES

ACL Tears

A Crabtree Forest Book

Crabtree Publishing
crabtreebooks.com

School-to-Home Support for Caregivers and Teachers

This appealing book is designed to teach students about core subject areas. Students will build upon what they already know about the subject and engage in topics that they want to learn more about. Here are a few guiding questions to help readers build comprehension skills. Possible answers appear here in red.

Before Reading:

- What do I know about ACL injuries?
  - *I know that ACL injuries happen in sports*
  - *I know that ACL injuries are knee injuries*
- What do I want to learn about this topic?
  - *I want to know how ACL injuries occur*
  - *I want to know how to prevent ACL injuries*

During Reading:

- I'm curious to know...
  - *I'm curious to know more about ACL anatomy*
  - *I'm curious to know if there are differences between boys and girls for ACL injuries*
- How is this like something I already know?
  - *I know that ACL injuries often happen in contact sports*
  - *I know that ACL injuries are common in sports*

After Reading:

- What was the author trying to teach me?
  - *The author was trying to teach me that there are many ways to treat ACL injuries*
  - *The author was trying to teach me that there are ways to help prevent ACL injuries*
- How did the photographs and captions help me understand more?
  - *The drawing of an ACL helped me understand its location in the body*
  - *The picture of an MRI machine helped me understand what might happen if I have an ACL injury*

Printed in the USA/

Table of Contents

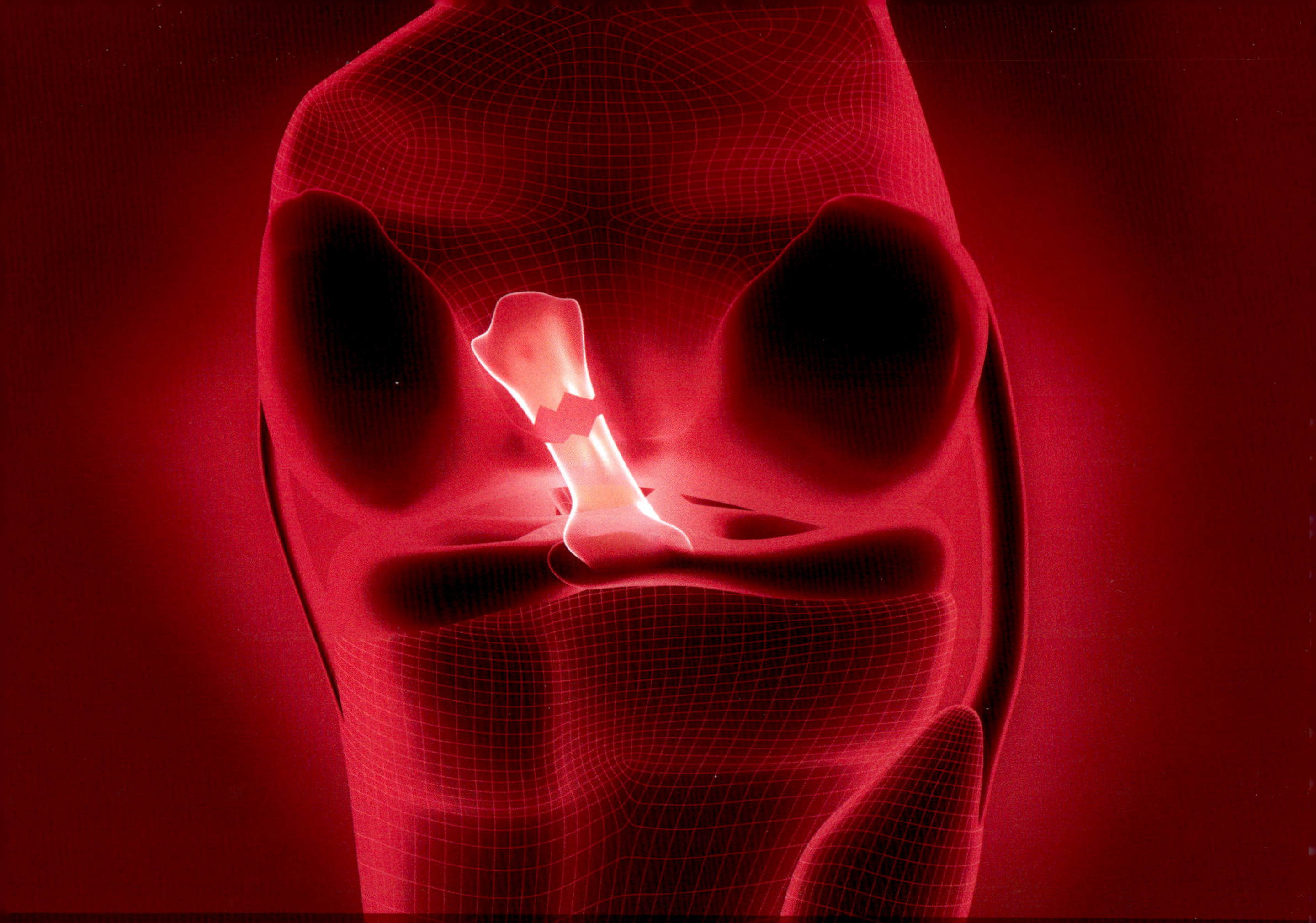

Chapter 1: What Are ACL Tears?

The skier races down the slope. Her skis glide over a box as she balances perfectly, her body twisting over the smooth surface. She dismounts and flies off the trick. But her skis land wrong. Her legs bend to absorb the force. She stops and clutches her knee. She's in too much pain to finish her run. What happened?

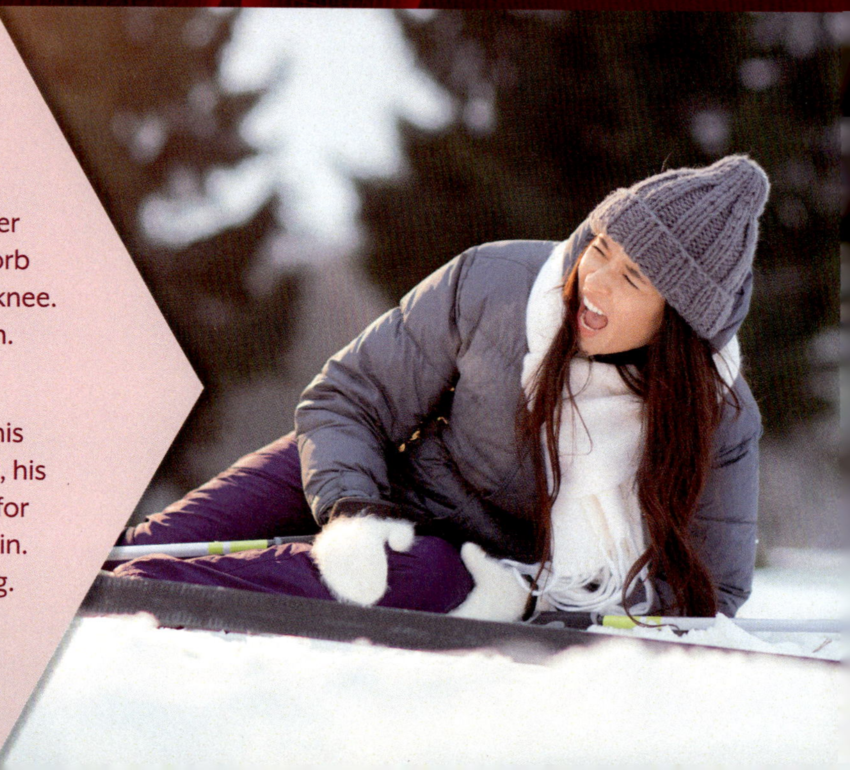

The soccer player stops the ball with his chest. As the ball drops to the ground, his right leg cuts behind his left to set up for a kick. But then, he doubles over in pain. He can't put any weight on his right leg. What happened?

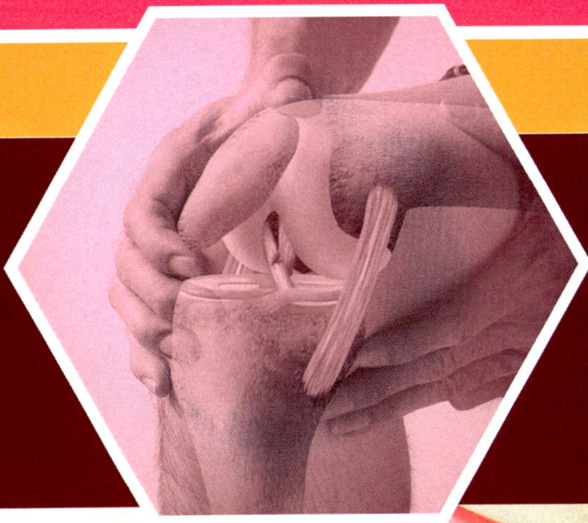

ACL Tears

These athletes both suffered ACL tears. ACL stands for **Anterior** Cruciate **Ligament**. It's one of the ligaments that hold the bones of your knee together. Without the ACL, your knee can't work properly. When your ACL is pulled too far or stretched in a direction it wasn't meant to go, it can tear.

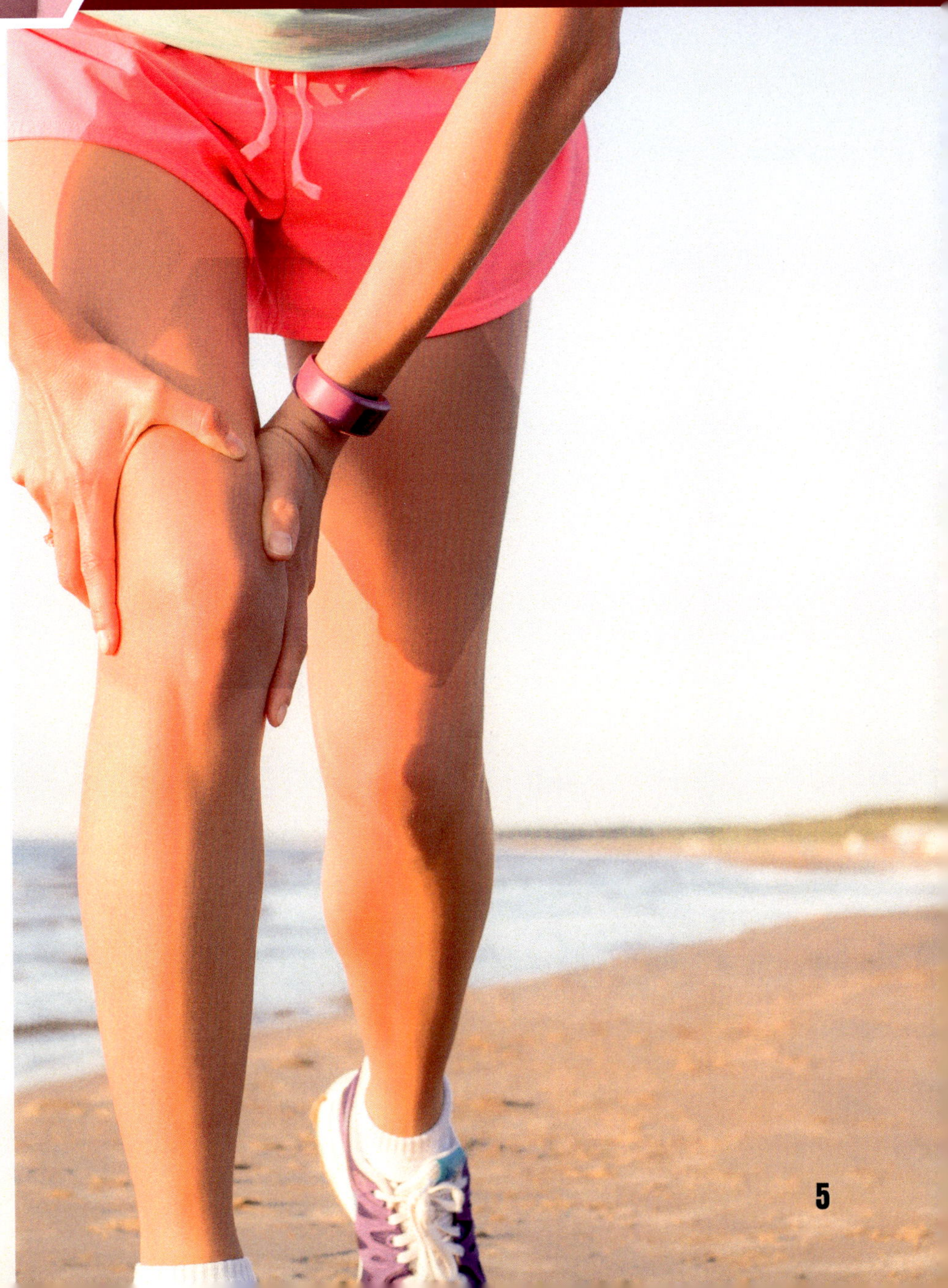

Sometimes people use the words "tendon" and "ligament" to mean the same thing, but they're actually different. Tendons connect ***muscle*** *to bone. Ligaments connect bones to other bones.*

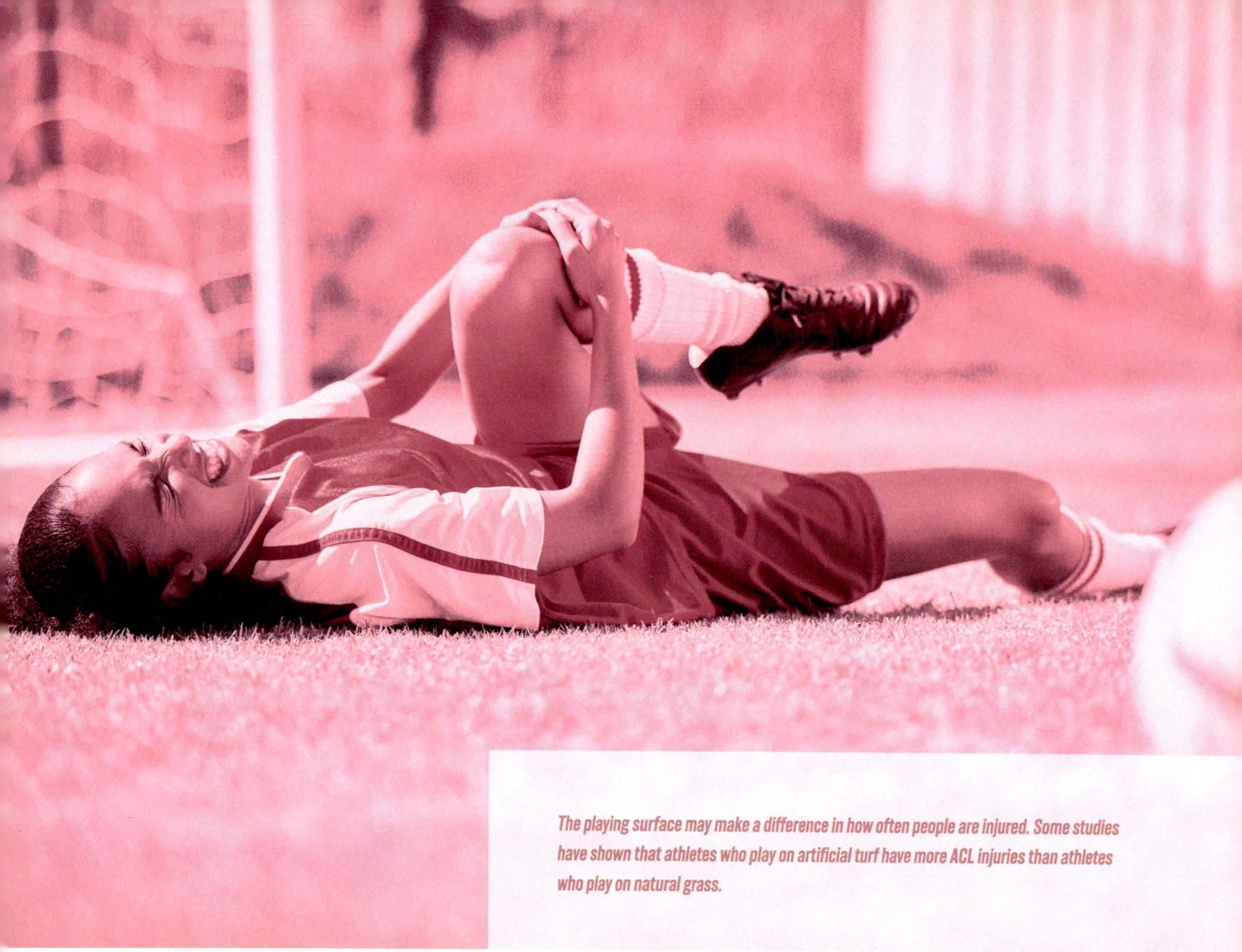

The playing surface may make a difference in how often people are injured. Some studies have shown that athletes who play on artificial turf have more ACL injuries than athletes who play on natural grass.

ACL tears are a common sports injury, both if you're playing for fun or playing professionally. There are as many as 200,000 ACL injuries in the United States every year. In the 2023 season, NFL players experienced 52 ACL tears. More than 25 female soccer players were benched during the 2023 World Cup because of ACL tears. Contact sports—such as basketball, soccer, and football—have many ACL tears, but any players of any sport that involves running and cutting can have this injury.

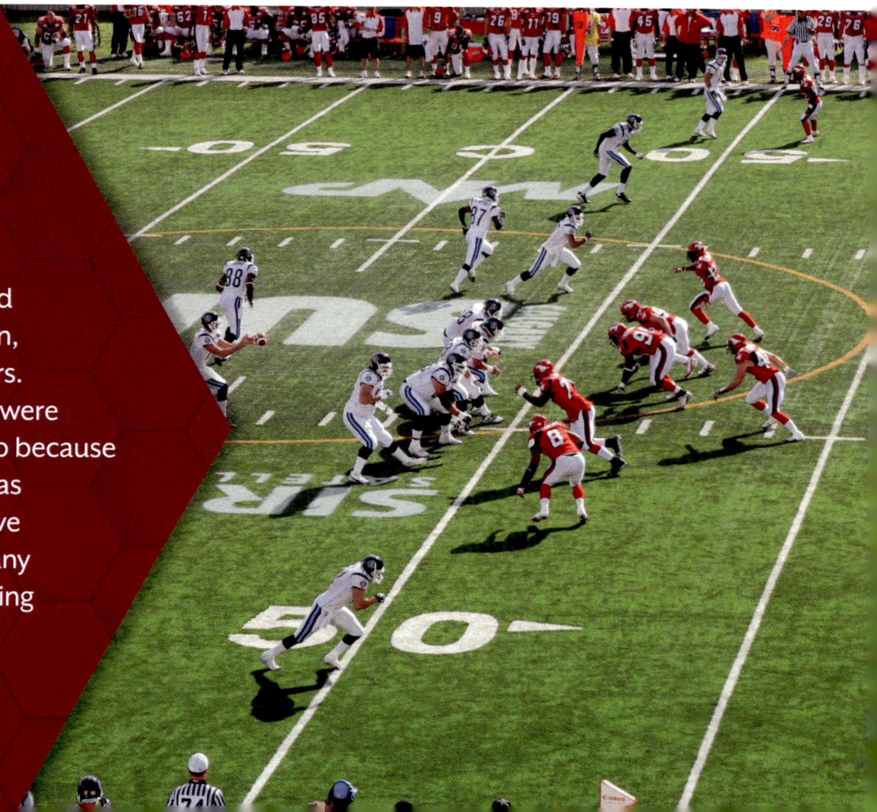

Many athletes suffer ACL tears, but there are ways you can help prevent this injury. When these injuries do occur, athletic trainers, doctors, and physical therapists have treatment plans to help you recover quickly. By learning about ACL **anatomy** and how ACL tears occur, you can work to keep your body heathy while playing sports.

Anatomy of the Knee

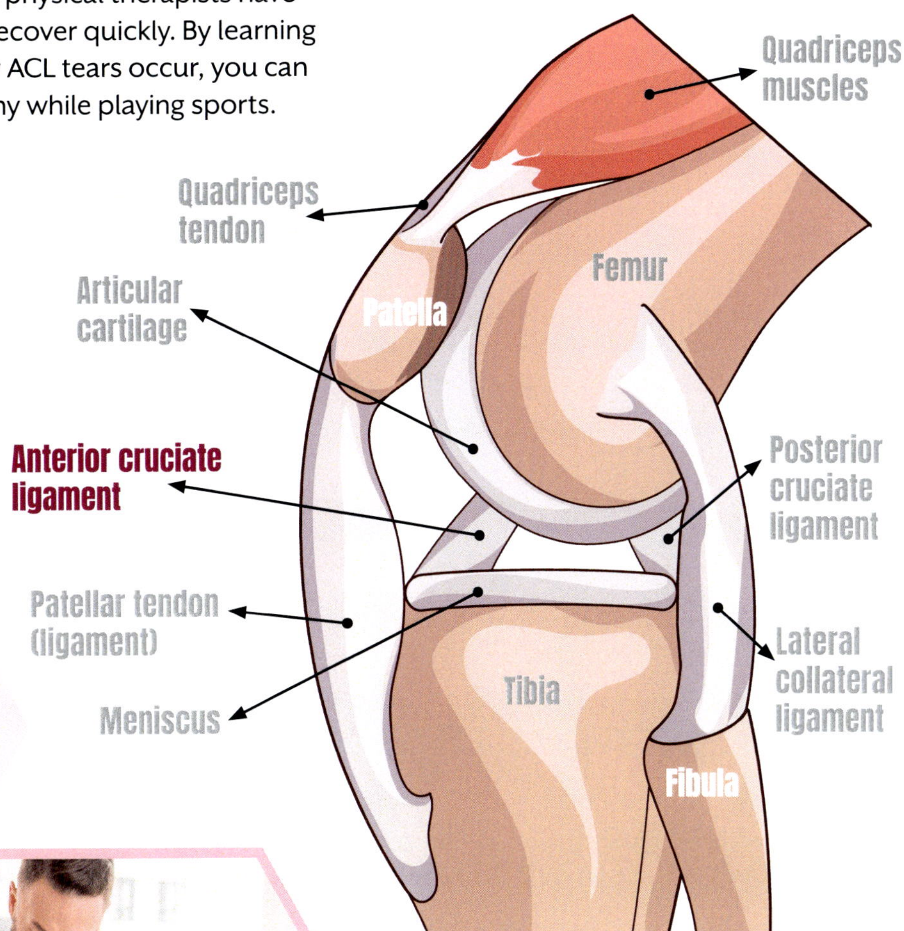

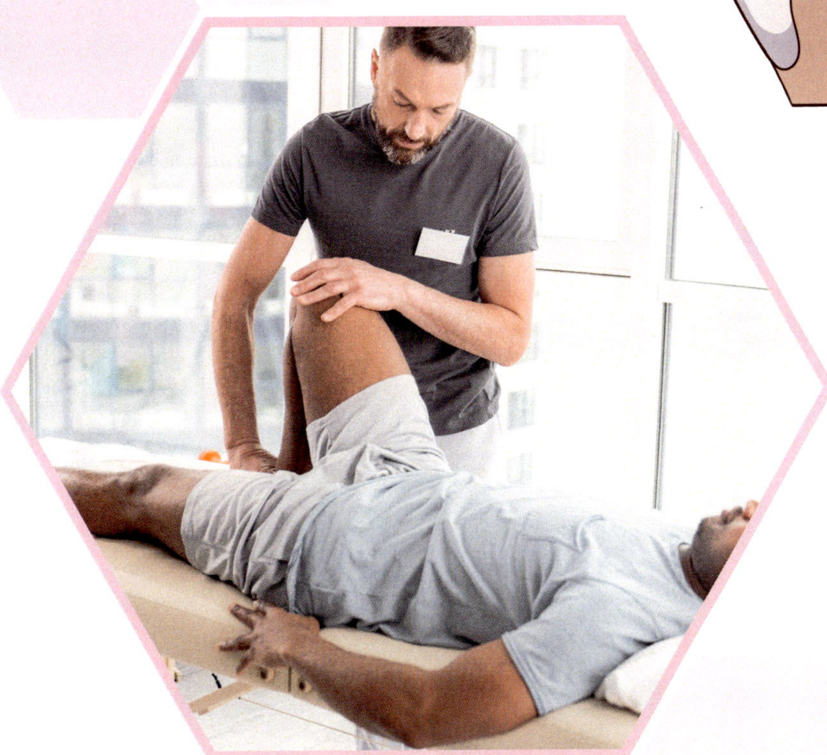

Chapter 2: Anatomy

Anatomy describes body parts and how they work together. Understanding how injuries happen starts with knowing the function of your muscles, bones, and ligaments.

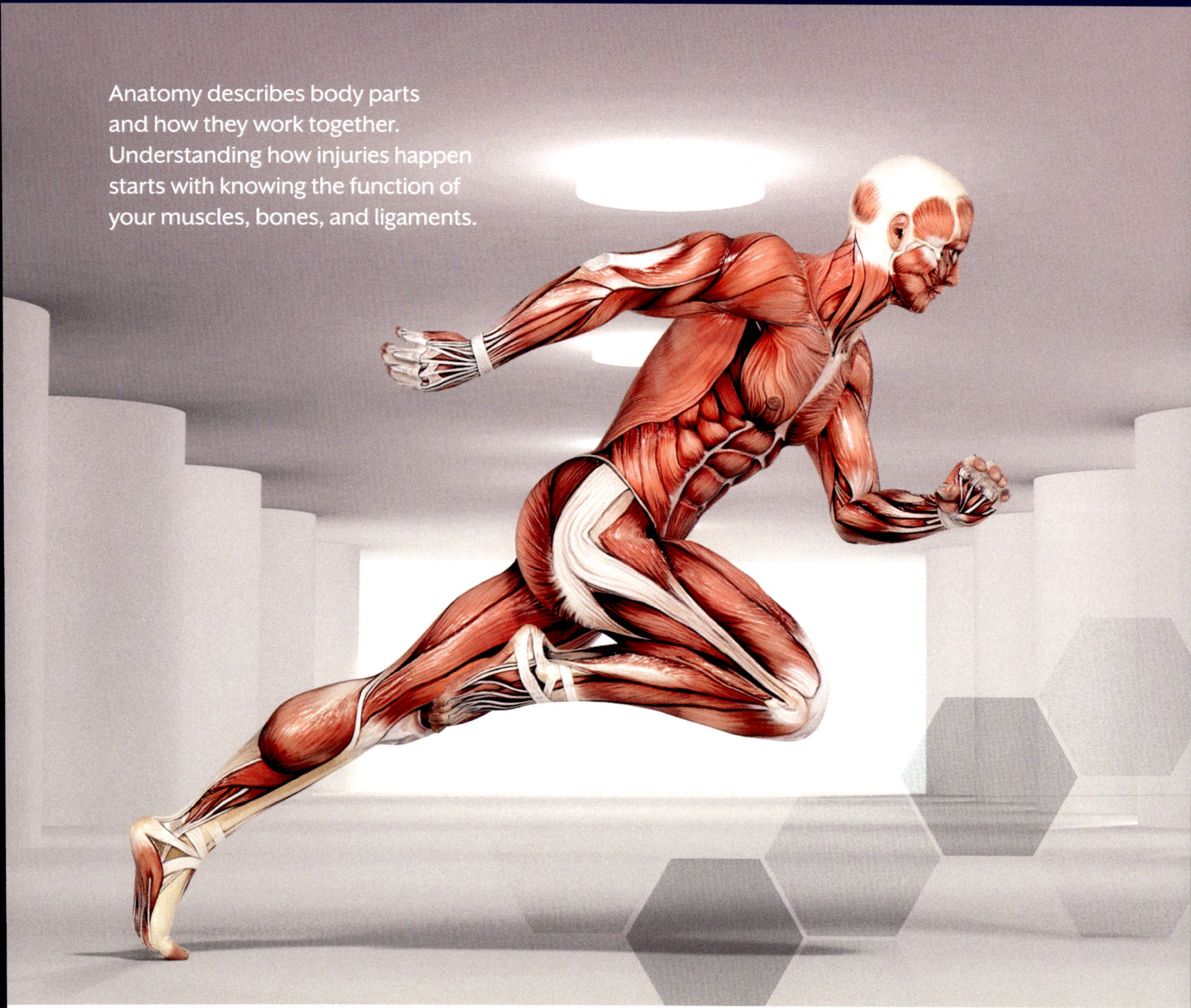

Bones

Hard bones support your body like a metal frame holds up a building. Some bones, such as your rib cage, also work to protect your soft organs.

Two bones play important parts in ACL injuries: your **femur** and your **tibia**. Your femur is the long bone of your upper leg. You might know it as the thigh bone. Your tibia is the shorter bone of your lower leg. It's sometimes called the shin bone.

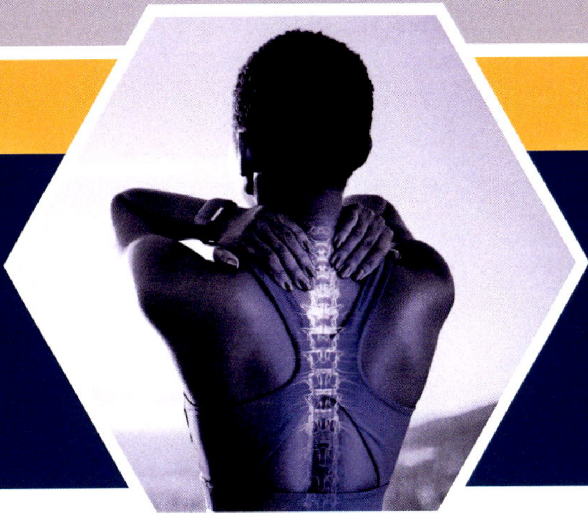

Joints

The place where two or more bones come together is called a joint. Some joints, like the bones of your skull, don't move. Other joints, like the bones of your spine, move just a little bit. However, many joints move a lot. These are called mobile joints.

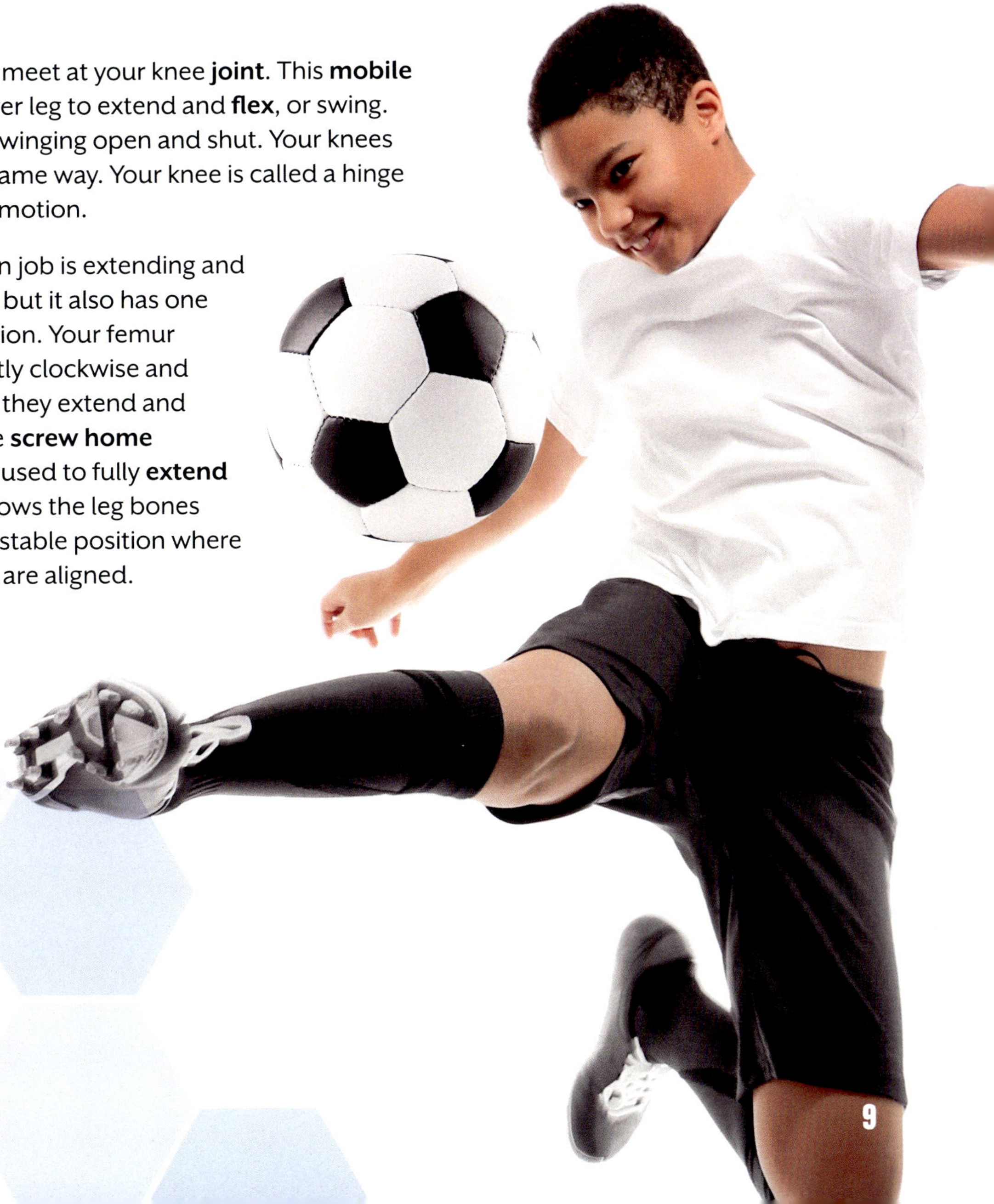

Your femur and tibia meet at your knee **joint**. This **mobile joint** allows your lower leg to extend and **flex**, or swing. Think about a door swinging open and shut. Your knees move in mostly the same way. Your knee is called a hinge joint because of this motion.

Your knee joint's main job is extending and flexing the lower leg, but it also has one more important motion. Your femur and tibia rotate slightly clockwise and counterclockwise as they extend and flex. This is called the **screw home mechanism**, and it's used to fully **extend** your leg. Rotating allows the leg bones to arrive at the most stable position where your femur and tibia are aligned.

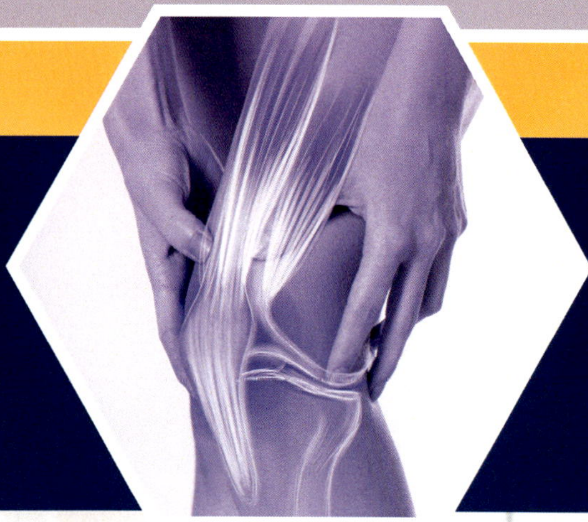

Ligaments

Ligaments are bands of tough, dense soft tissue that connect bones and organs to help hold them in place. Think of them like strong ropes. You have over 900 ligaments in your body! Four ligaments in the knee connect the femur to the tibia. They work to keep your upper and lower leg aligned.

The femur is the longest bone in your body. The bones inside your ear– the hammer, anvil, and stirrup – are the shortest.

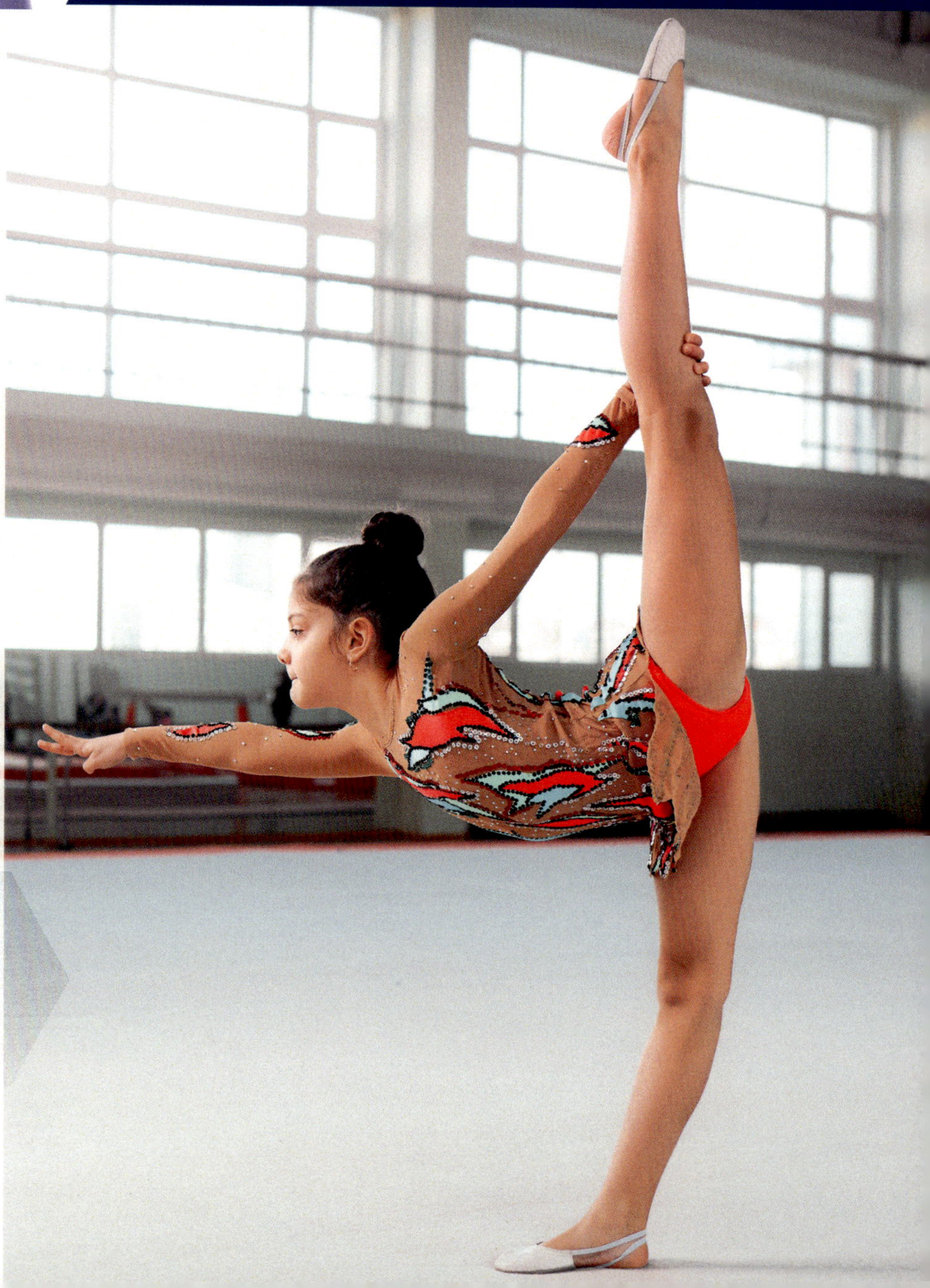

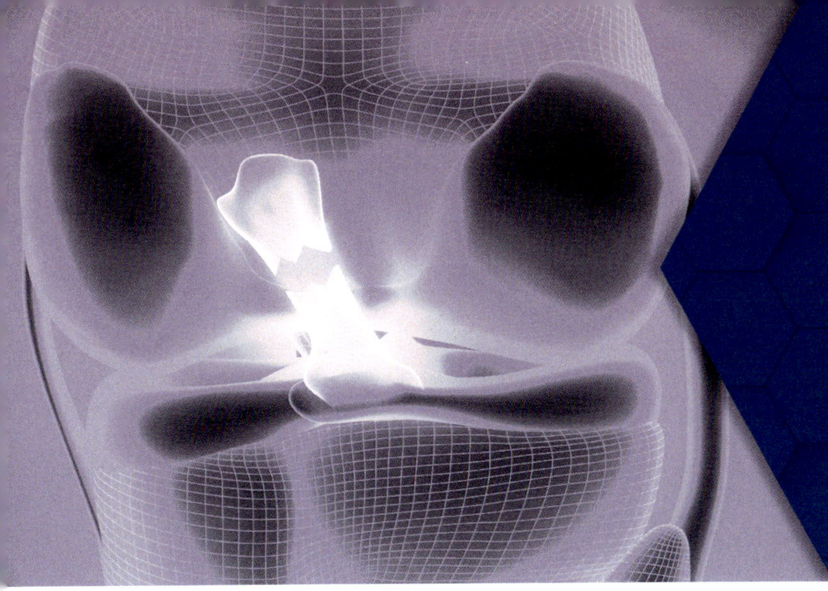

The Anterior Cruciate Ligament (ACL) is in the front of your knee. Anterior is the anatomical word for front.

Cruciate means "to cross." The ACL gets its name, because it looks like it makes an X, or crosses, with the Posterior Cruciate Ligament just behind it. These ligaments work with your other knee ligaments to help control leg motion and to keep your knee stable.

Your ACL is a small ligament. It's only about 1 to 1.5 inches (27 to 38 mm) long. It looks like an hourglass; the widest part attaches to the bone.

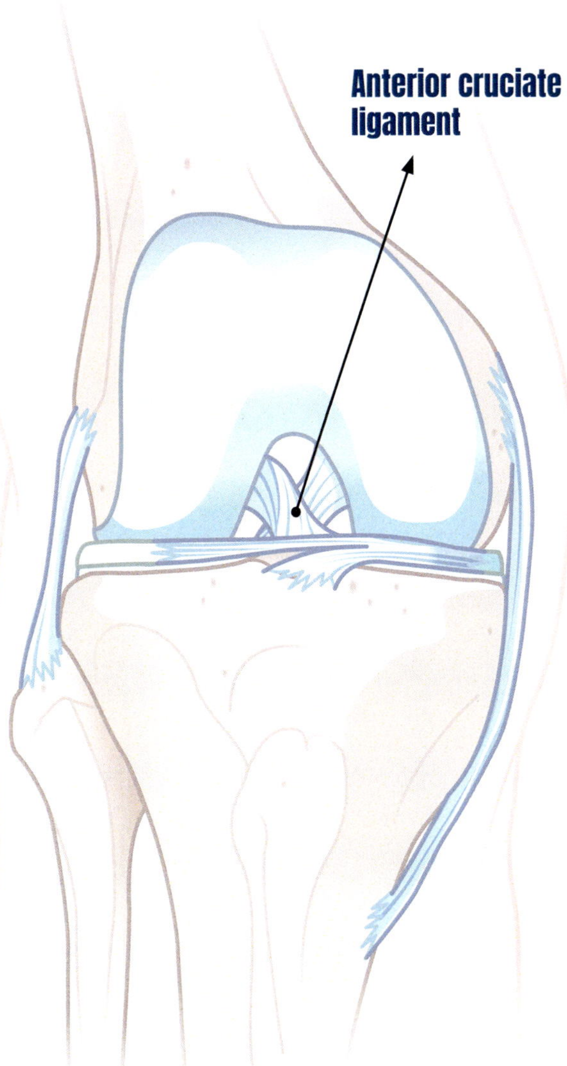

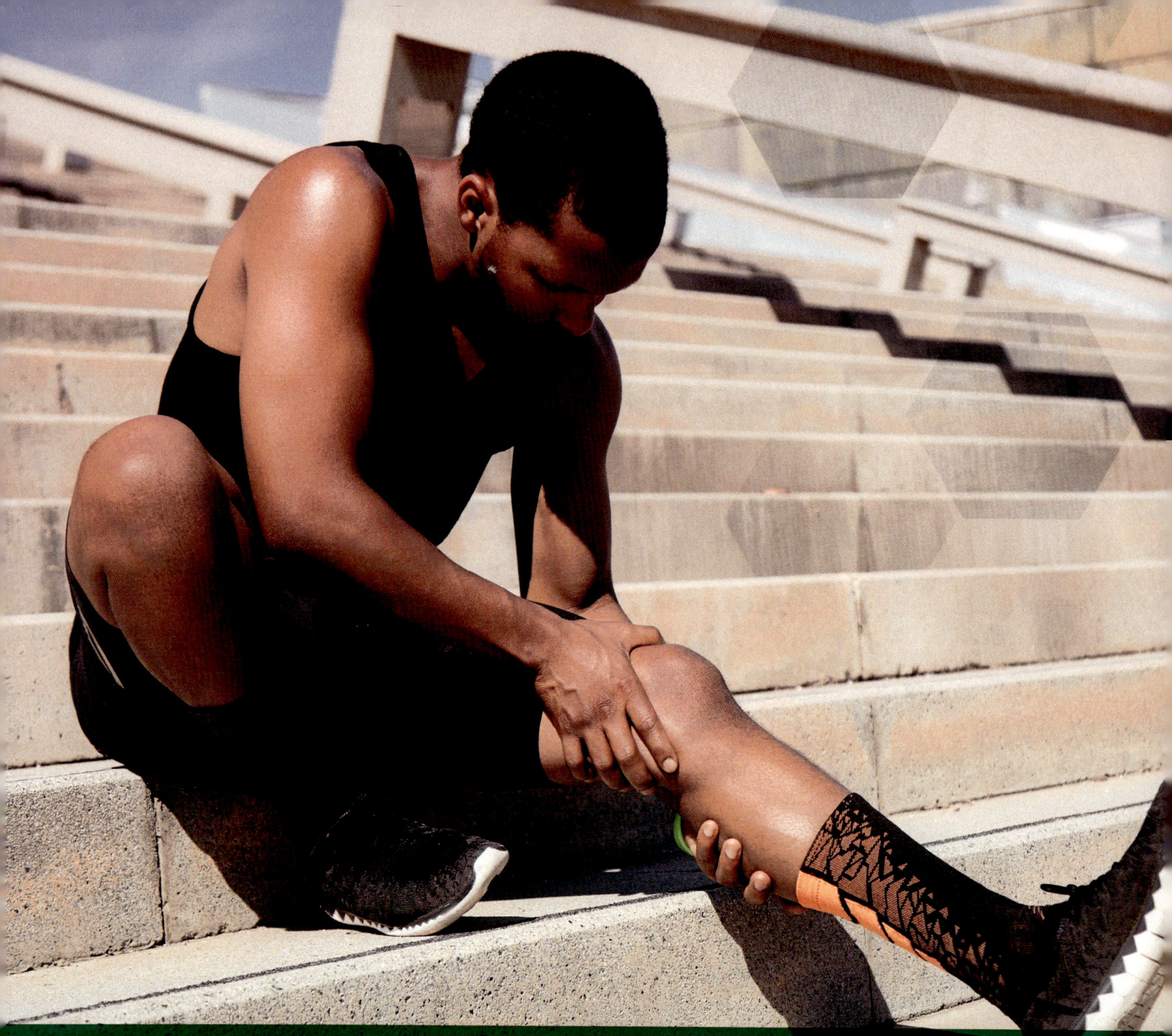

Chapter 3: Causes of ACL Injuries

Stretching your ACL too far can cause it to suddenly tear. This is called an acute injury. This term means that the tear happened all at once instead of slowly over time.

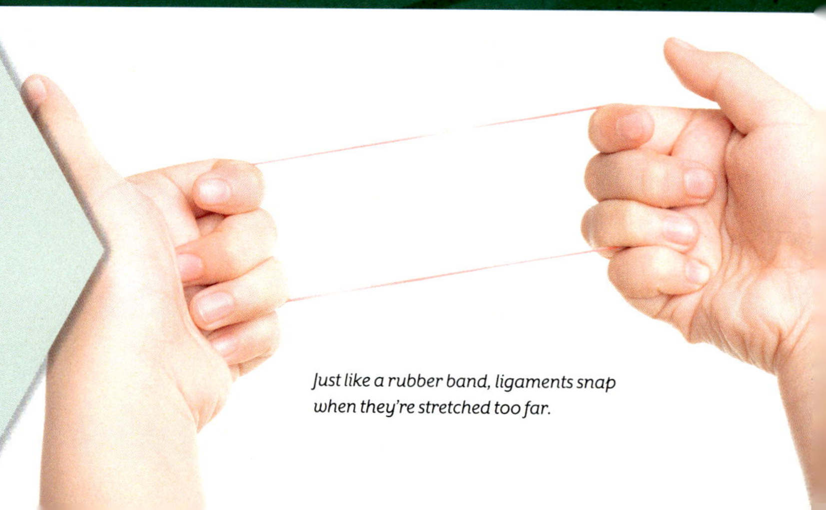

Just like a rubber band, ligaments snap when they're stretched too far.

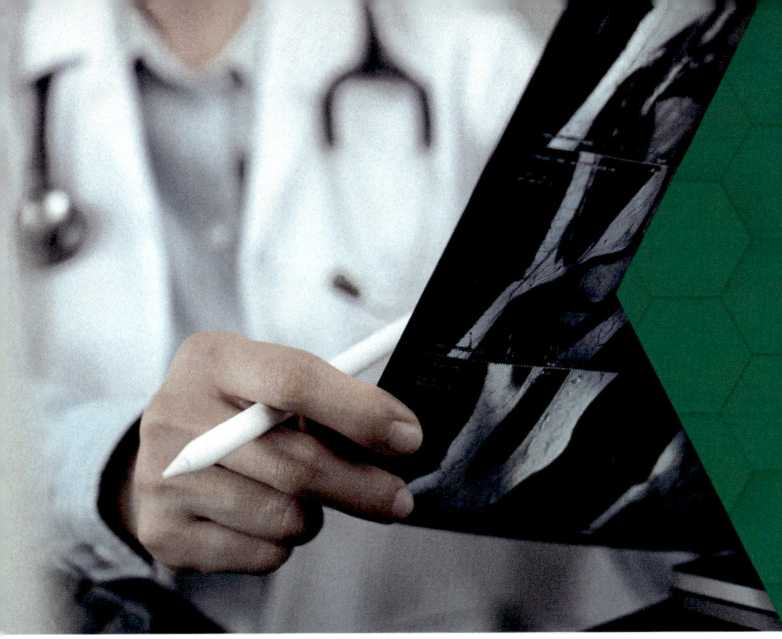

Doctors and scientists study ACL injuries to find out what causes the ligament to tear. They've found that certain motions are more likely to result in injuries. Some of these motions are

- Stopping or slowing down suddenly
- Changing direction (cutting) too fast
- Landing incorrectly from a jump
- Blunt force from outside of the knee

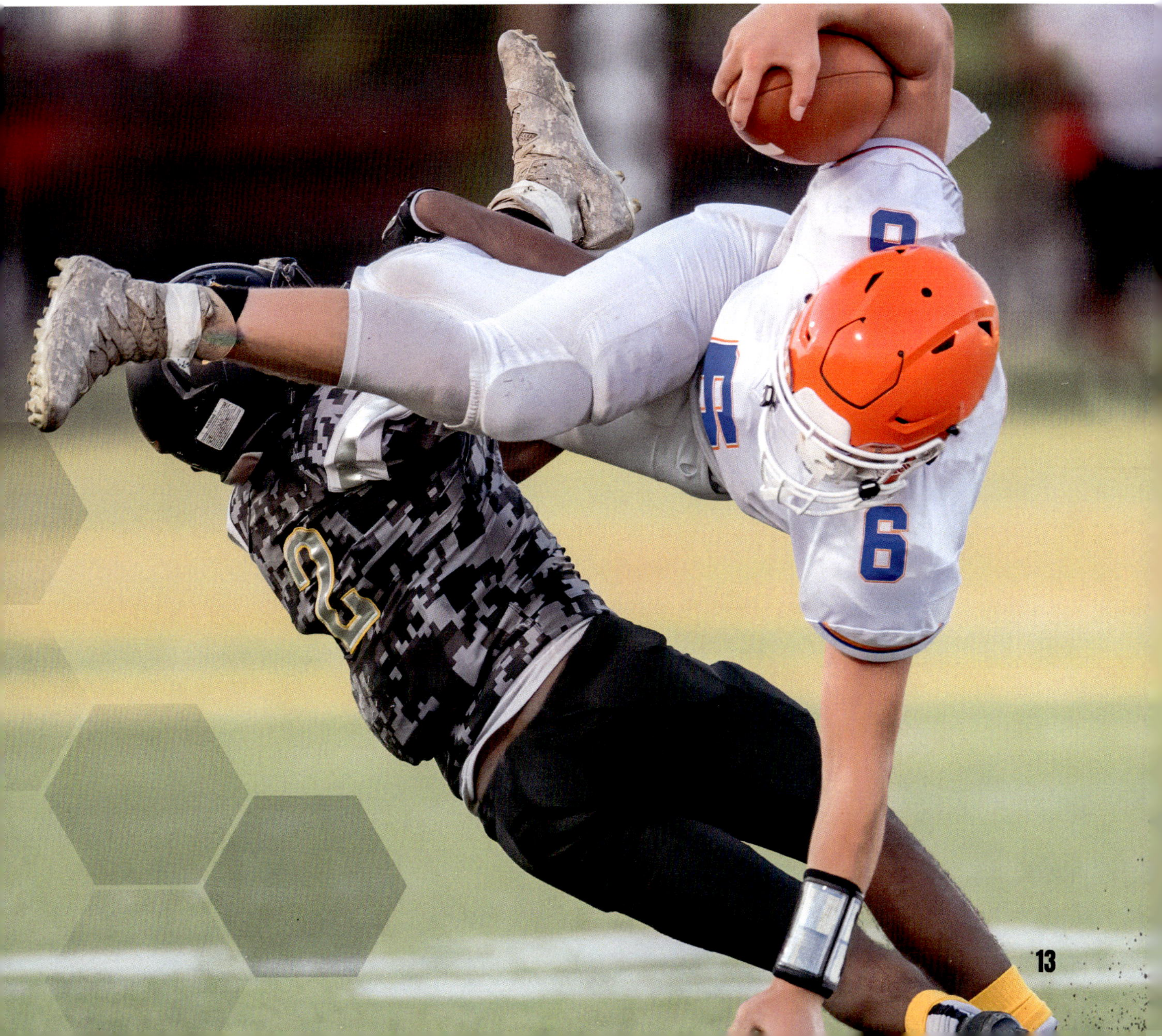

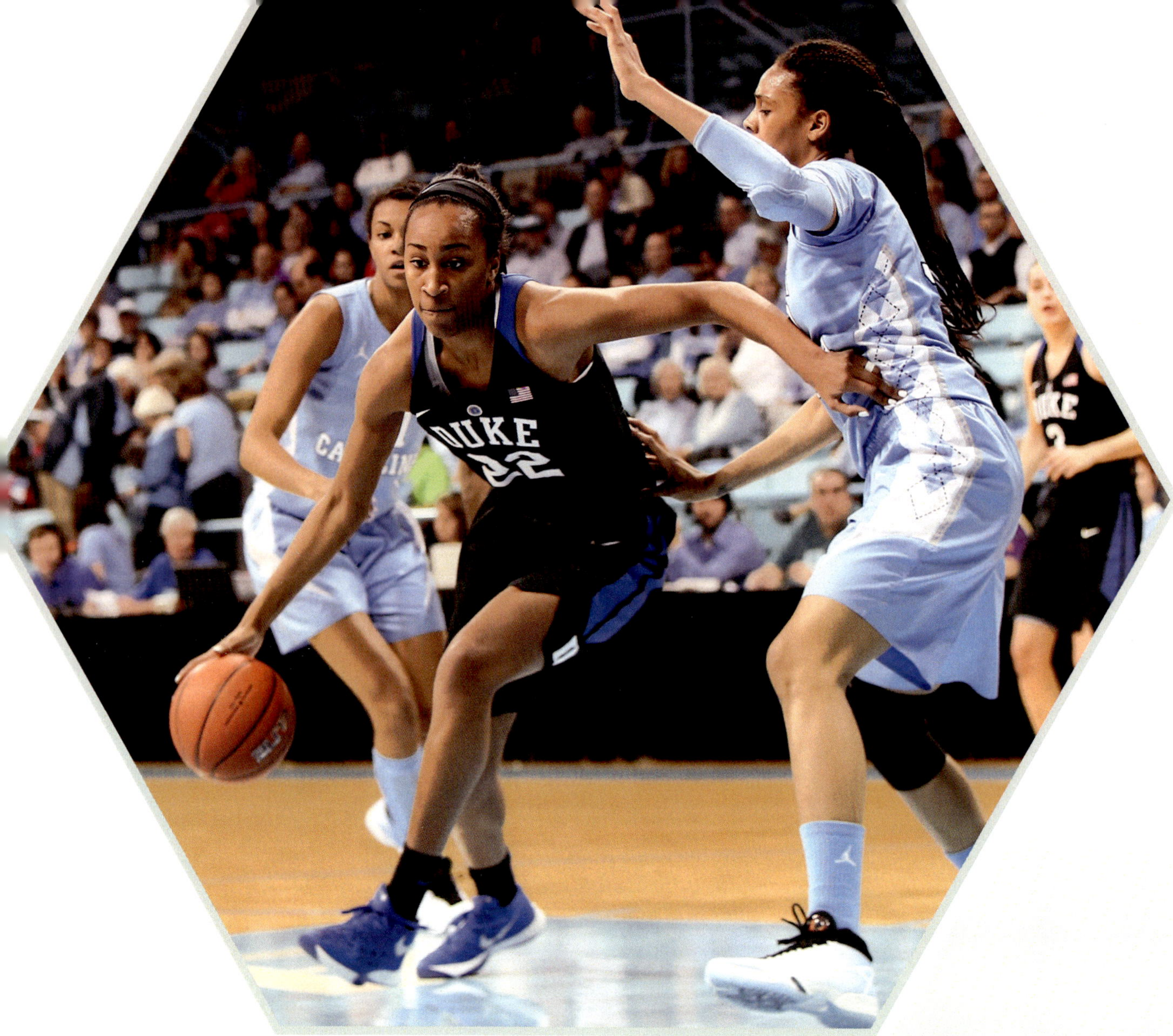

It's easy to see why ACL tears are so common in sports. Stopping and starting suddenly, changing direction quickly, and jumping are all motions that athletes perform every day. These motions are especially common in sports like football, basketball, and soccer. Athletes who play these sports are known to have a lot of ACL tears.

Being tackled also causes ACL tears. When blunt force is applied to the knee – like when a linebacker sacks the quarterback – the ACL can tear. This can also happen anytime one athlete runs into another, such as during soccer and basketball games. Outside of sports, workplace accidents and car crashes are also times when an ACL injury can occur in a similar way.

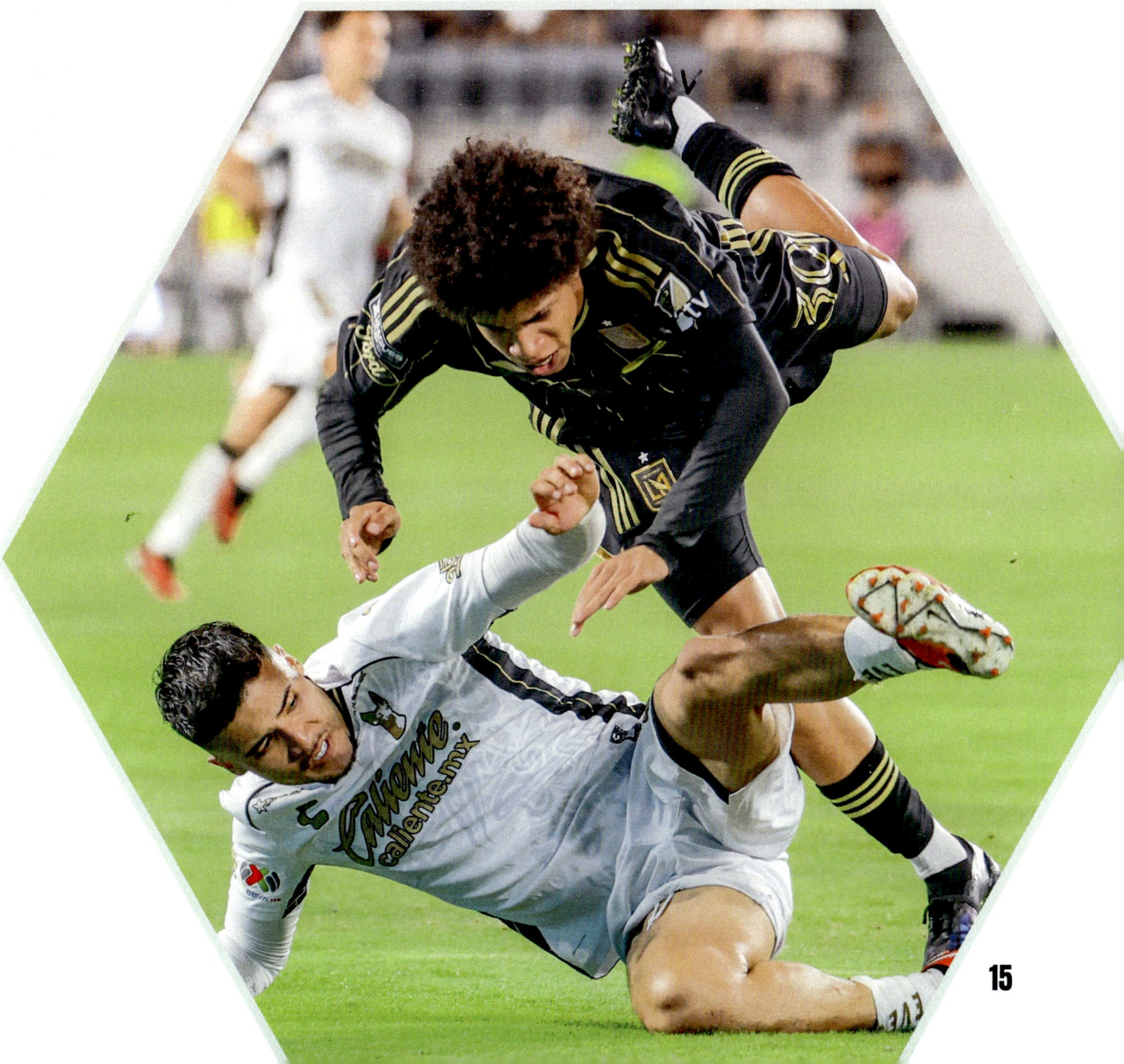

ACL Injuries in Female Athletes

Women and girls are more likely to experience an ACL tear than men. In fact, women and girls are two to eight times more likely to experience an ACL tear than men. Doctors and scientists aren't entirely certain why there's a difference in injuries between women and men, but they have some hypotheses.

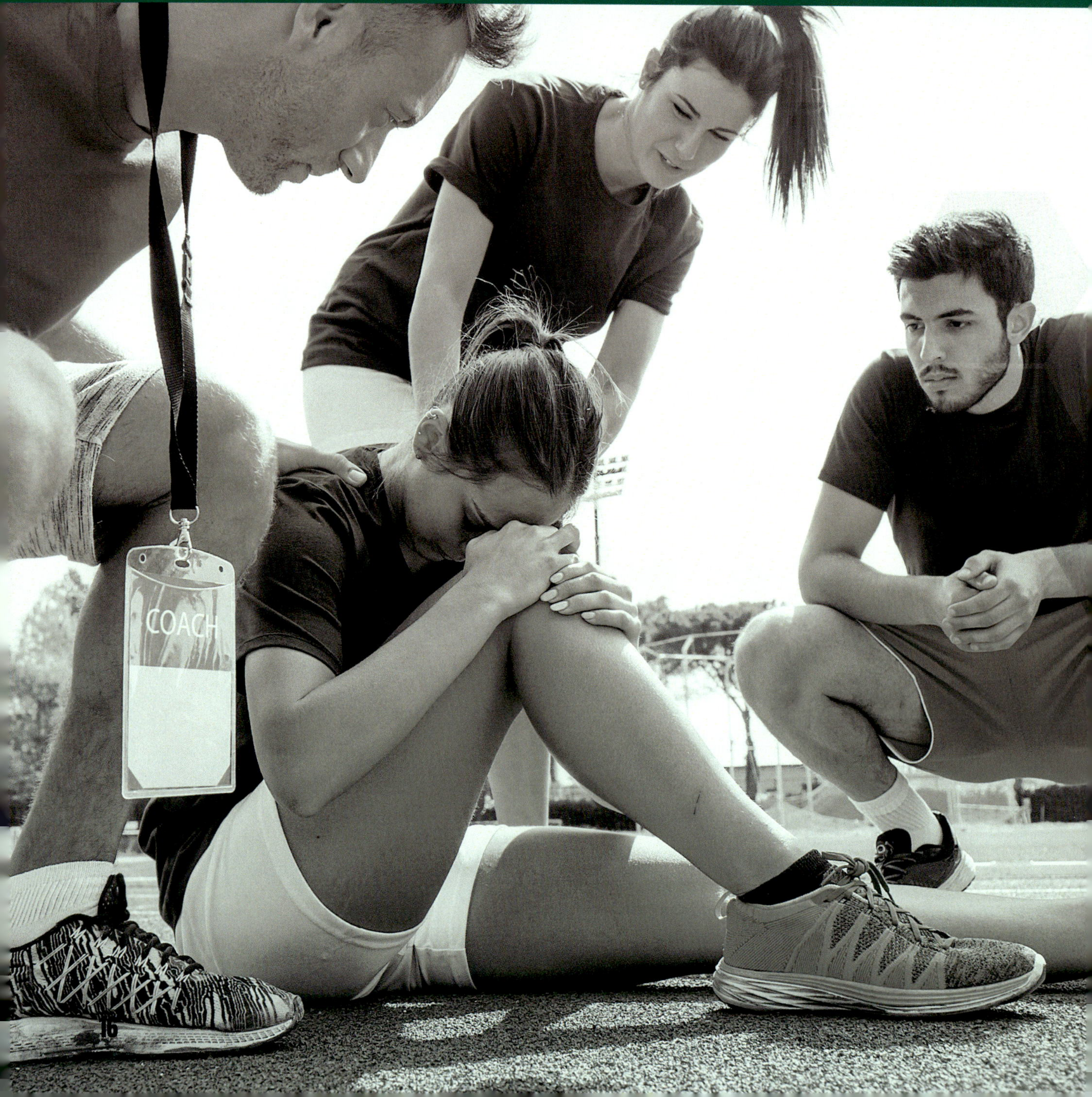

Biomechanical engineers play an important role in understanding sports injuries. They use knowledge of physics, or the study of matter and forces, and apply it to the human body. Biomechanical engineers use information like how pelvis shape is different between men and women to design equipment to keep athletes safe.

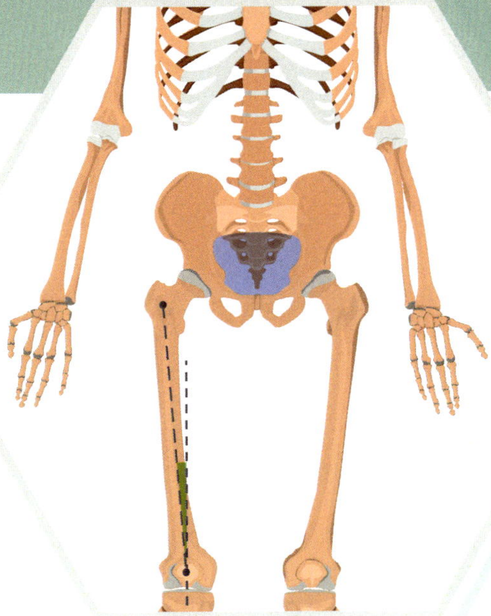

Male Pelvis

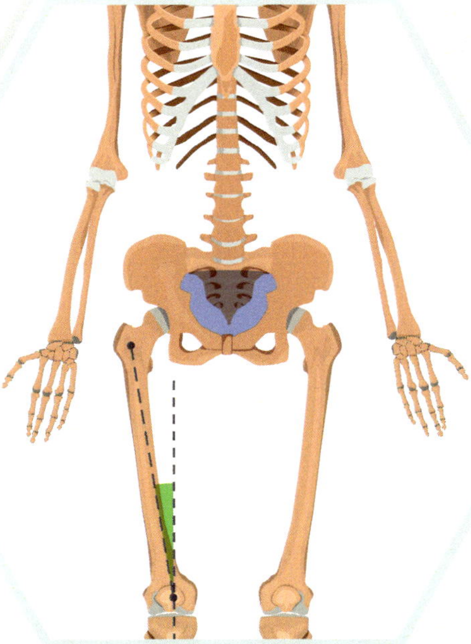

Female Pelvis

One **hypothesis** is that female ACL injuries happen often because the female **pelvis** is wider than a male pelvis. This means that the female femur is at a different angle to the tibia than in. It may mean that there is more stress on the ligaments of a female knee than on a male knee.

Another hypothesis is that women and men also have different amounts of muscle around their knees. Muscle, along with ligaments, helps to keep the knee joint stable. Because women have less muscle mass than men, their knees might be less stable, which makes the ACL more likely to be injured.

Hormones are also different between men and women, and that's another hypothesis about ACL injuries. These chemicals influence everything from muscle density to how tight or loose ligaments are. This means that **hormones** may play a part in how stable the knee joint is.

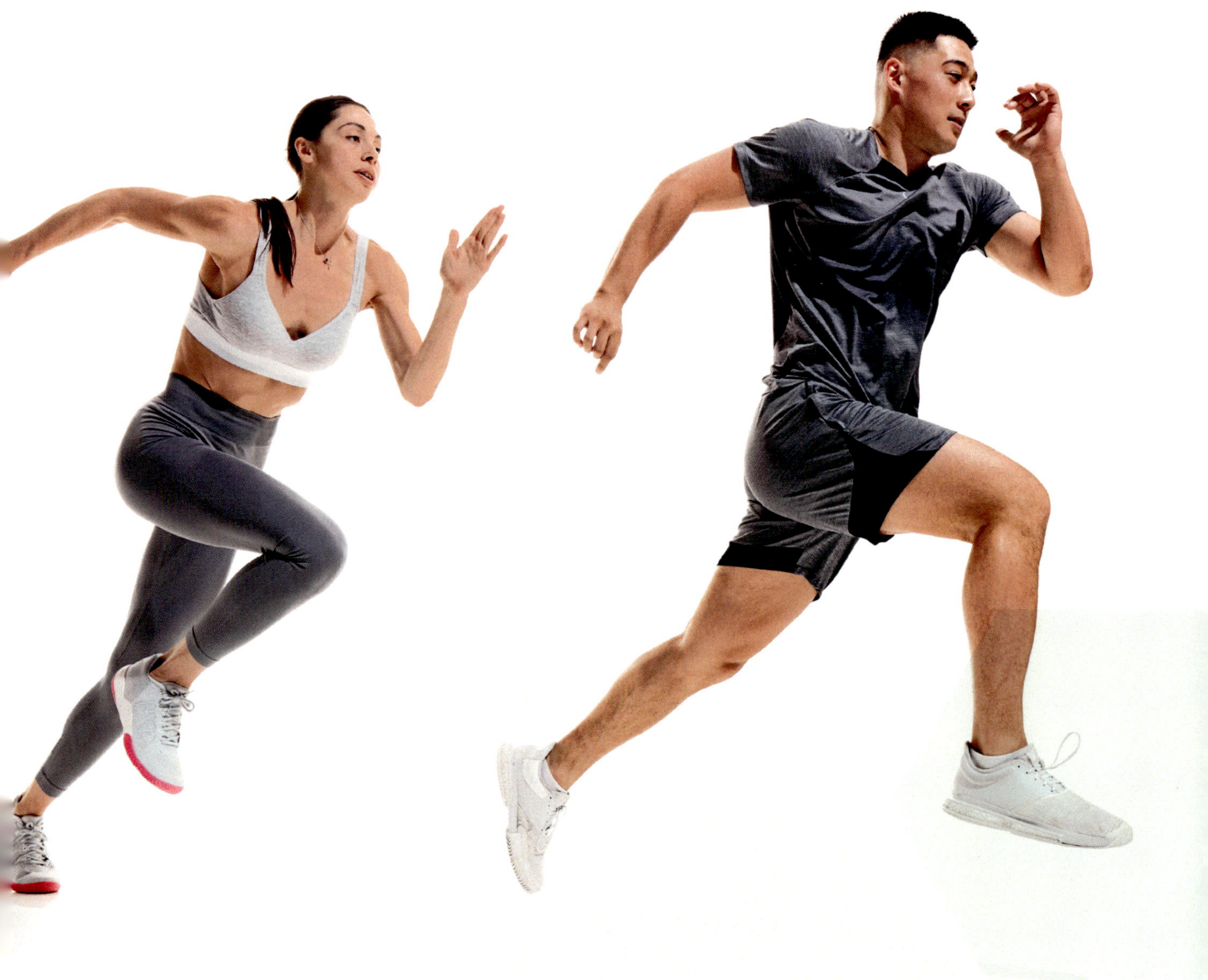

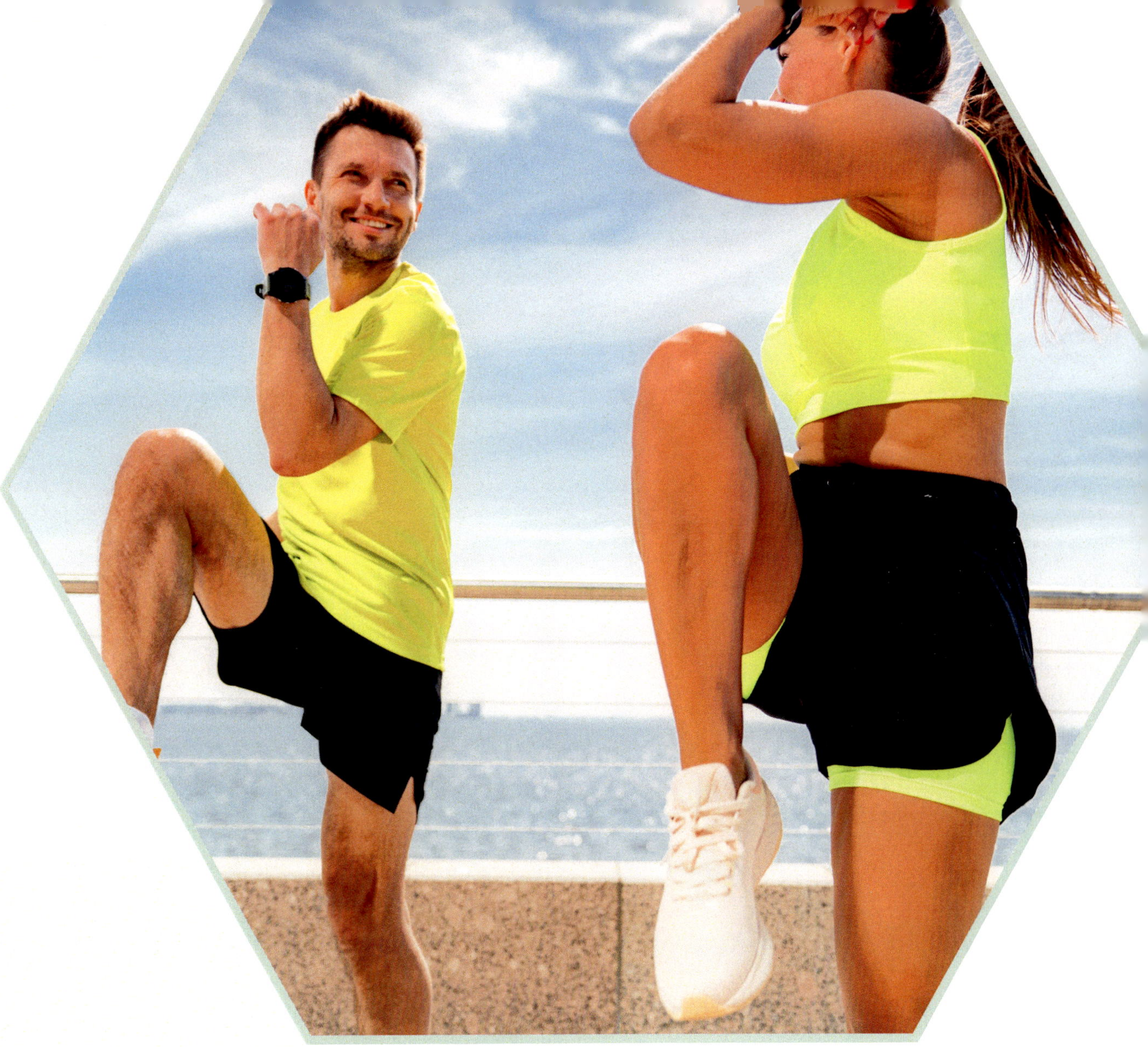

Scientists and doctors are still working to understand how these different elements influence injury. Is one more important than the others? How do pelvis shape, muscle tone, and hormones work together to influence how likely an athlete is to be injured? These are all good questions, and more research is needed to understand the differences in ACL injuries between women and men.

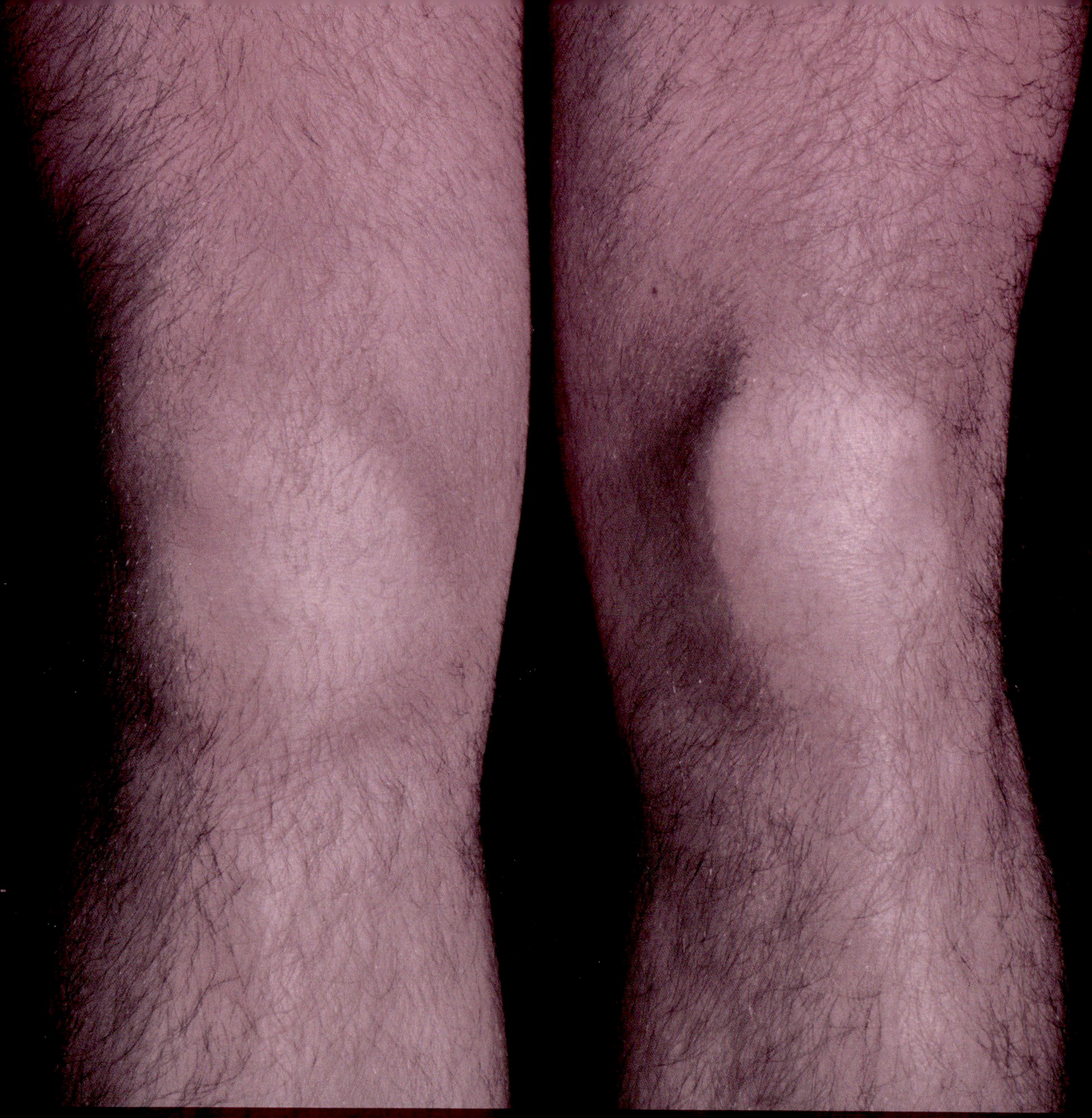

Chapter 4: Types of ACL Tears

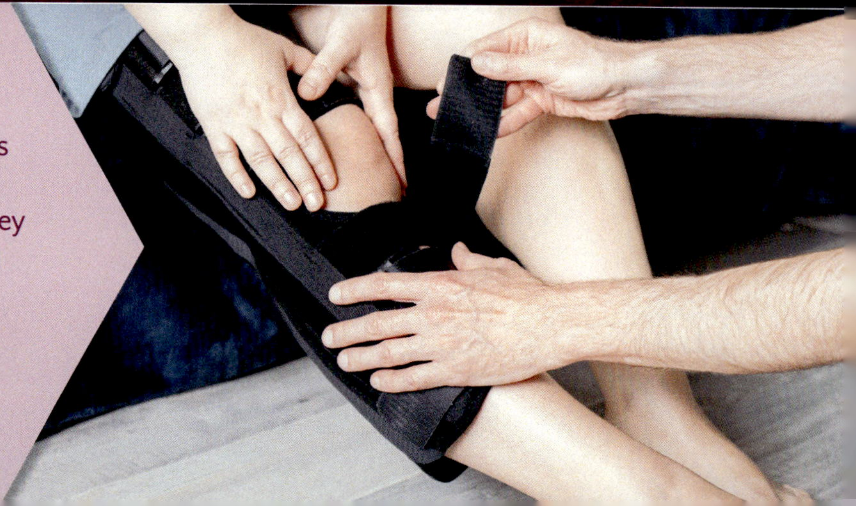

ACL injuries can range from just a small ligament strain to a complete tear. Doctors and medical professionals have developed a grading system to help identify how badly you're hurt. They use this grading system to recommend treatment.

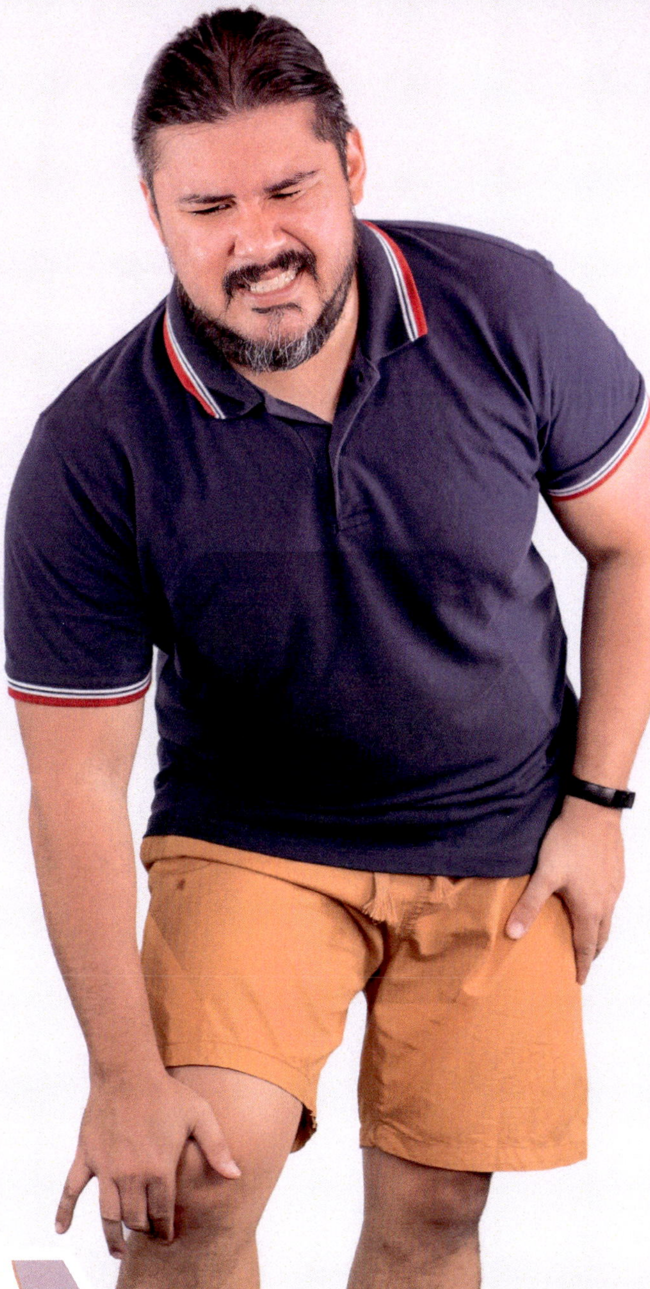

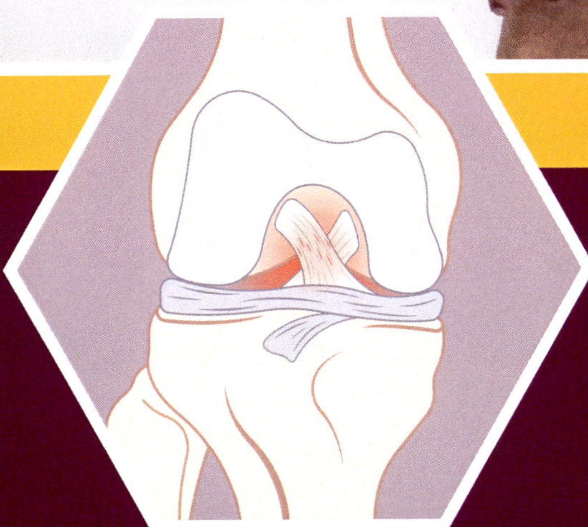

Grade 1

Grade 1 ACL injuries are the least severe. These are usually called ligament strain injuries. If there are tears, they're so small that it takes a microscope to see them. If you have a Grade 1 injury, you'll feel some pain around your knee, but your leg can hold weight to stand. You will likely still be able to walk.

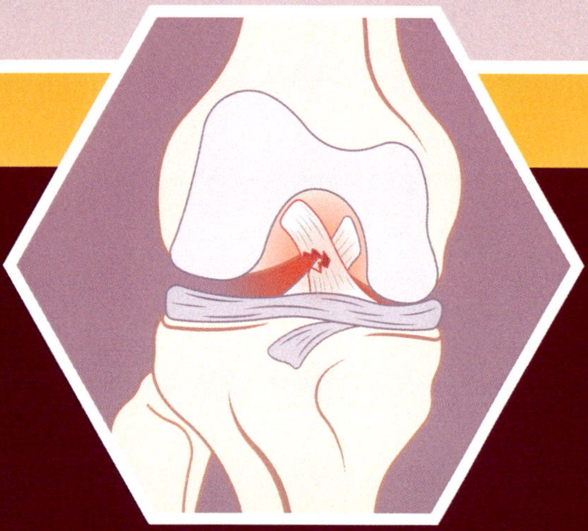

Grade 2

Grade 2 ACL injuries are the most uncommon. If you have a Grade 2 injury, you have tears through 20-80 percent of the ACL. The tears are more visible than in Grade 1, but you're still able to stand and possibly move. Unfortunately, the pain in a Grade 2 injury is also greater than in a Grade 1 injury. You will have noticeable bruising and swelling. While you may be able to move, your knee may look wobbly.

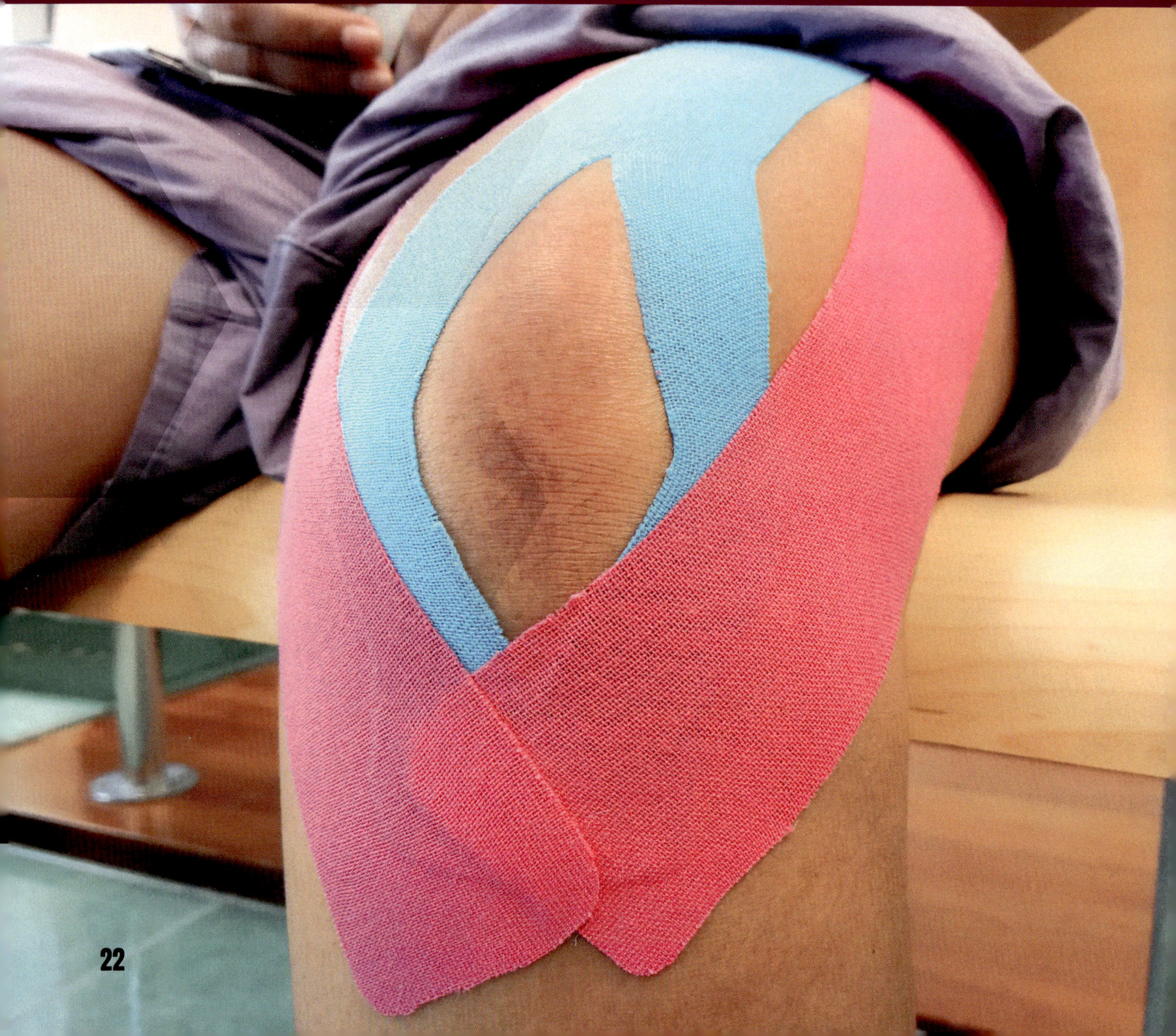

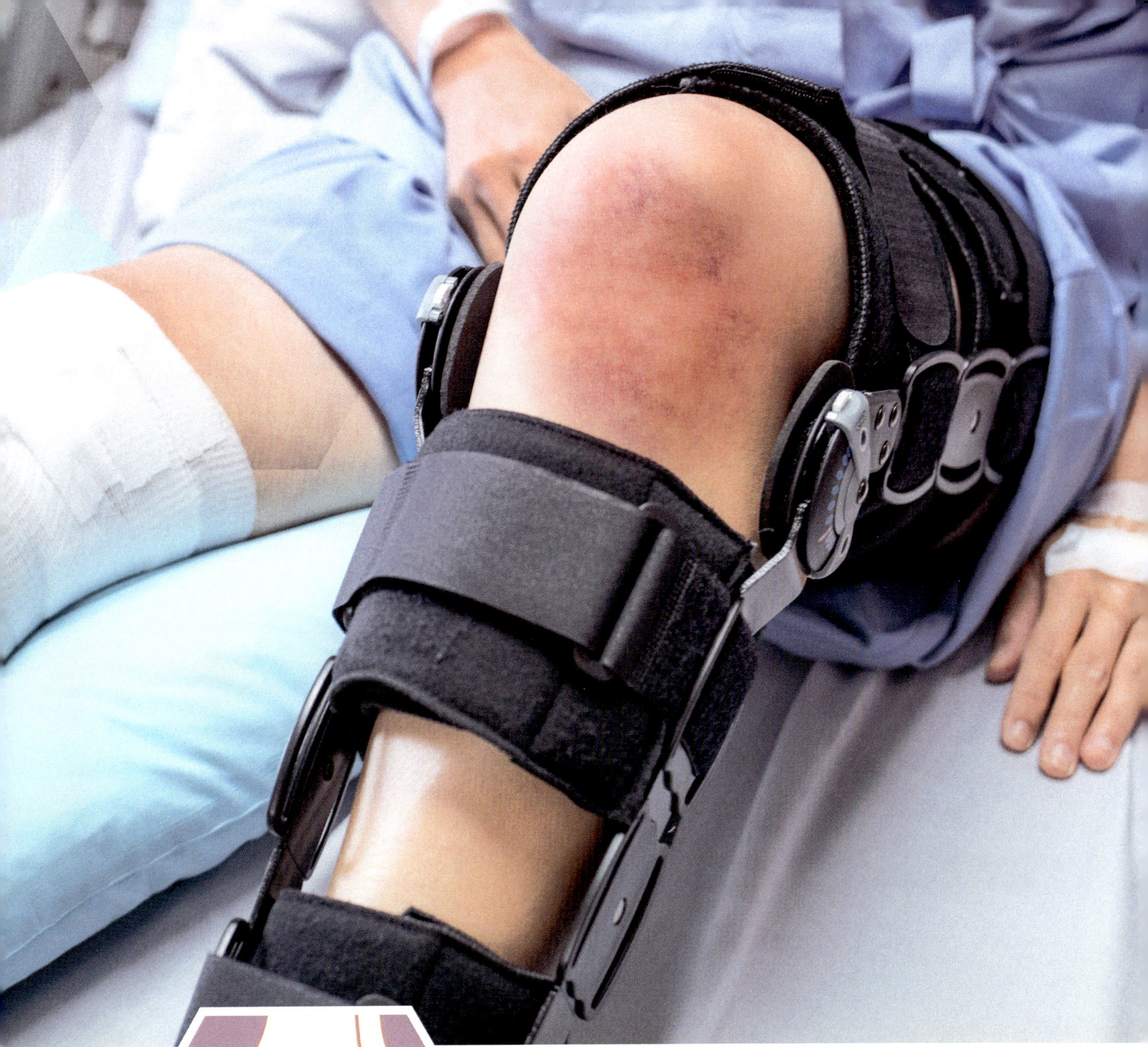

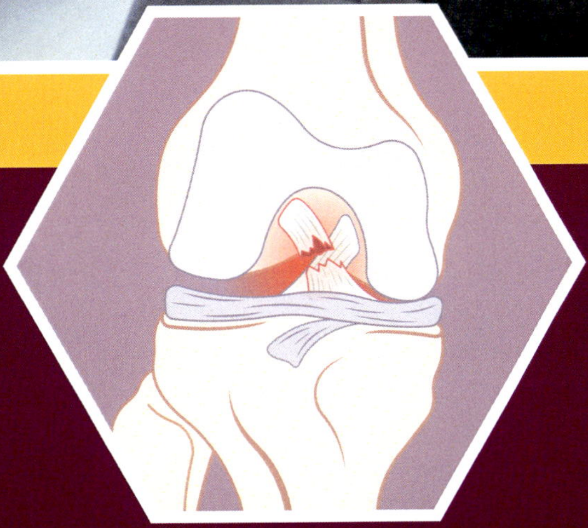

Grade 3

Grade 3 ACL injuries happen when you completely tear the ligament. Often you will hear a "snap" or "pop" noise and feel the moment when the ligament ruptures. You'll no longer be able to move your knee or put any weight on it. This is because your ACL ligament is no longer attached and is in two separate pieces, so it can't keep the femur and tibia in the right place.

Avulsion Injury

Avulsion ACL injuries usually only occur in youth athletes. Sometimes when you injure your ACL, your ligament does not tear. Instead, your ACL will break away from your tibia with some of the bone still attached to the ligament. This is called an **avulsion injury**.

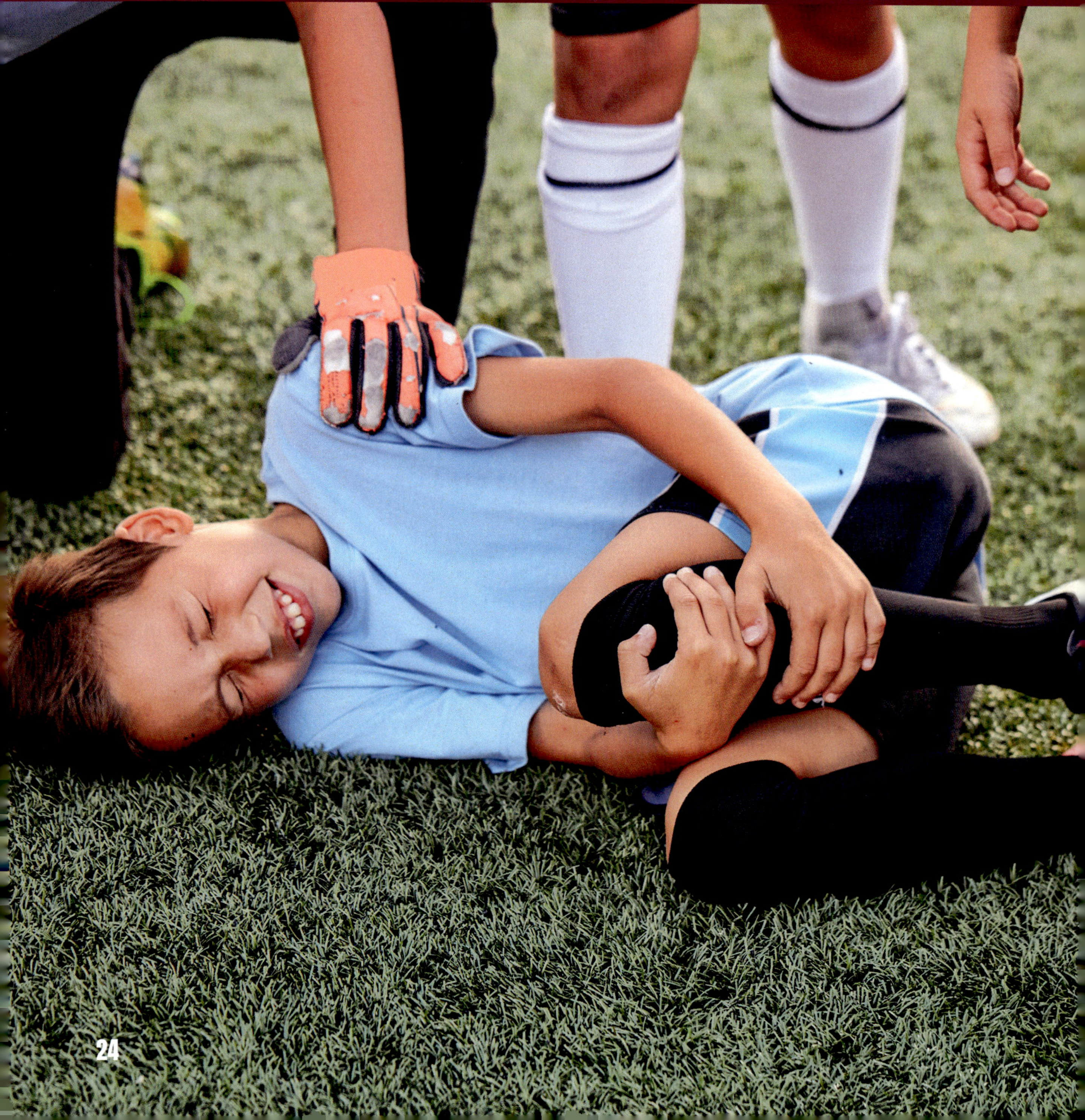

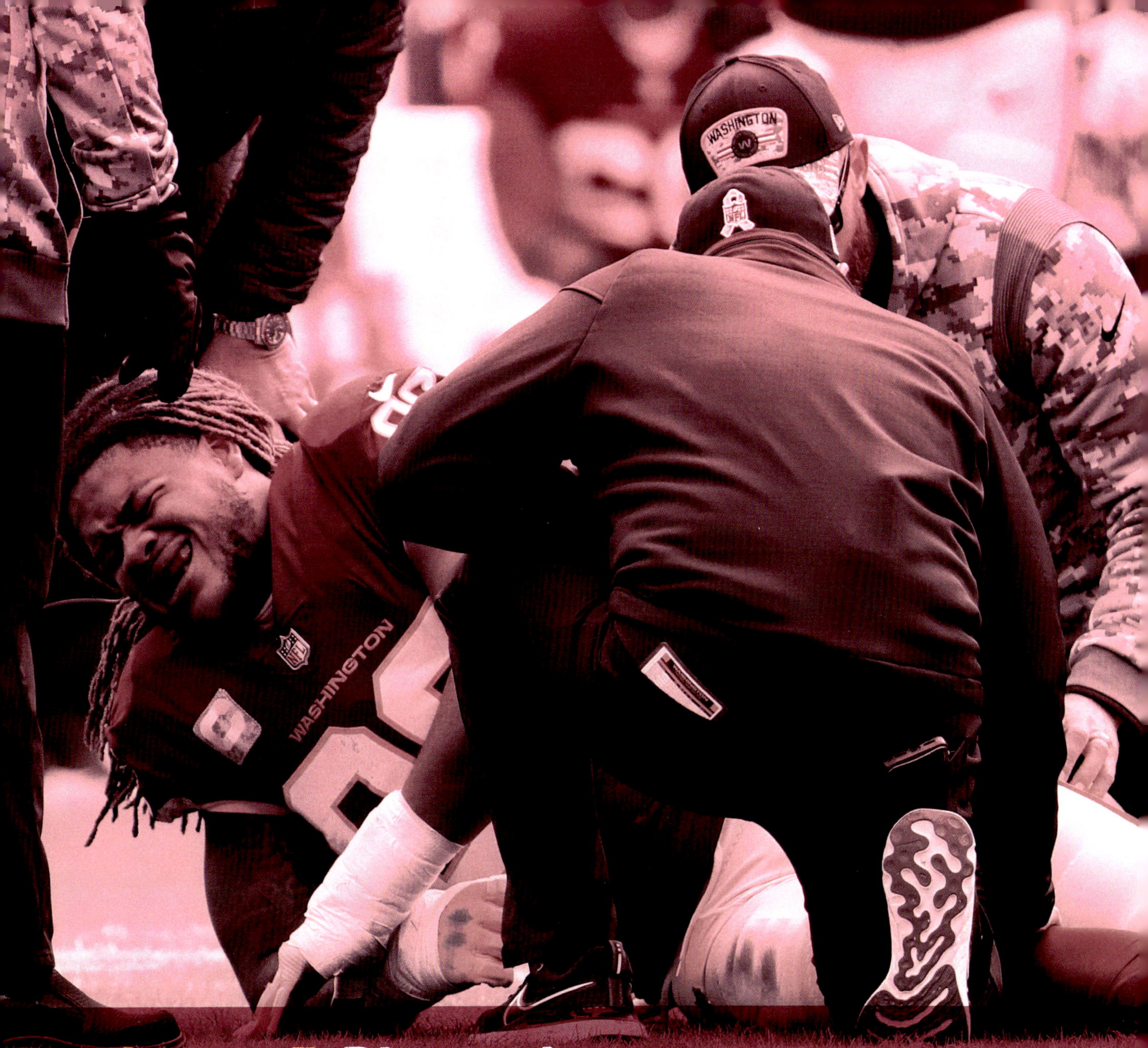

Chapter 5: Diagnosis

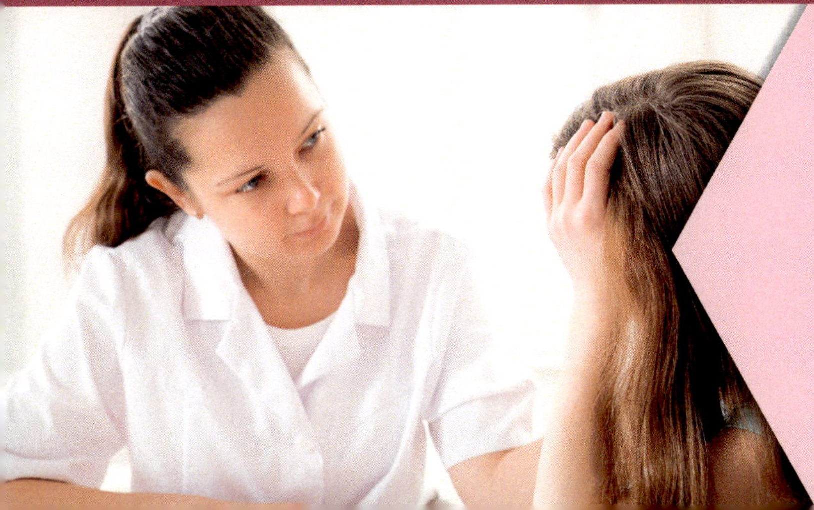

You will notice when you have an ACL injury. Even with a mild, Grade 1 injury, you will feel pain. For more severe injuries, game play or practice may have to be stopped in order to help the injured athlete or to help you off the field.

You should see a medical professional as soon as you're injured. Athletic trainers may be the closest medical personnel to you, and they can help you reach a doctor. Only medical professionals are able to diagnose an ACL tear and create a plan for your treatment and recovery.

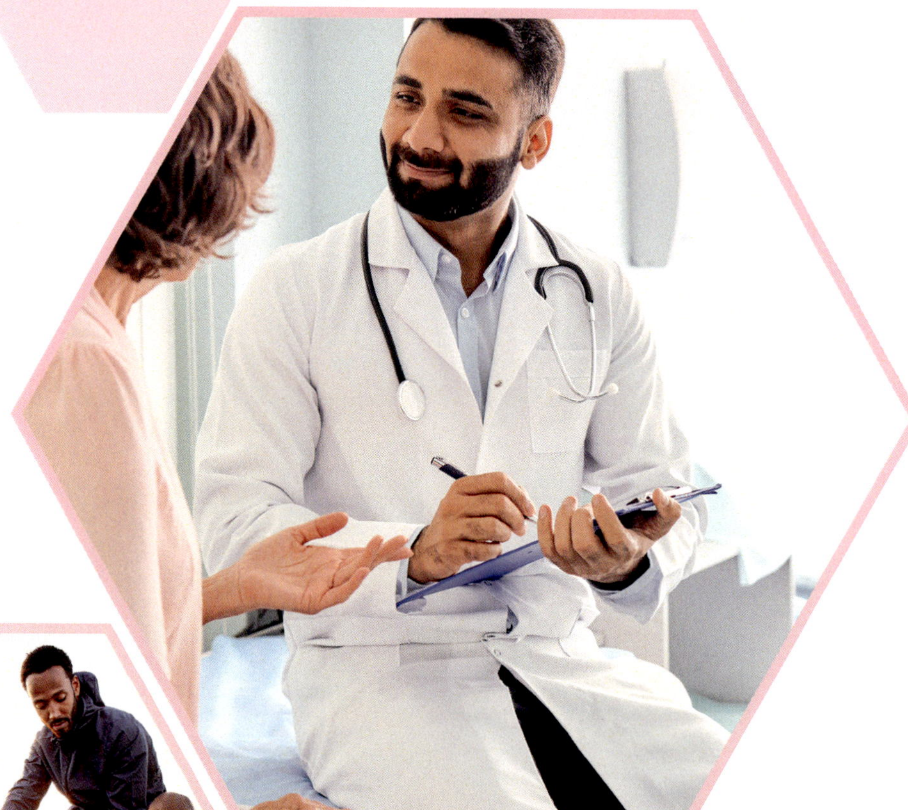

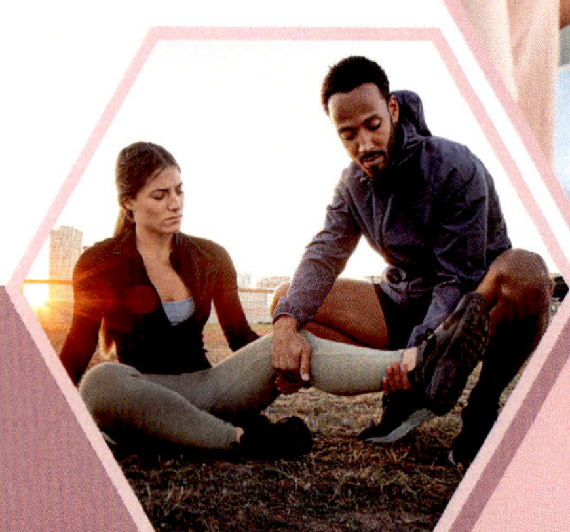

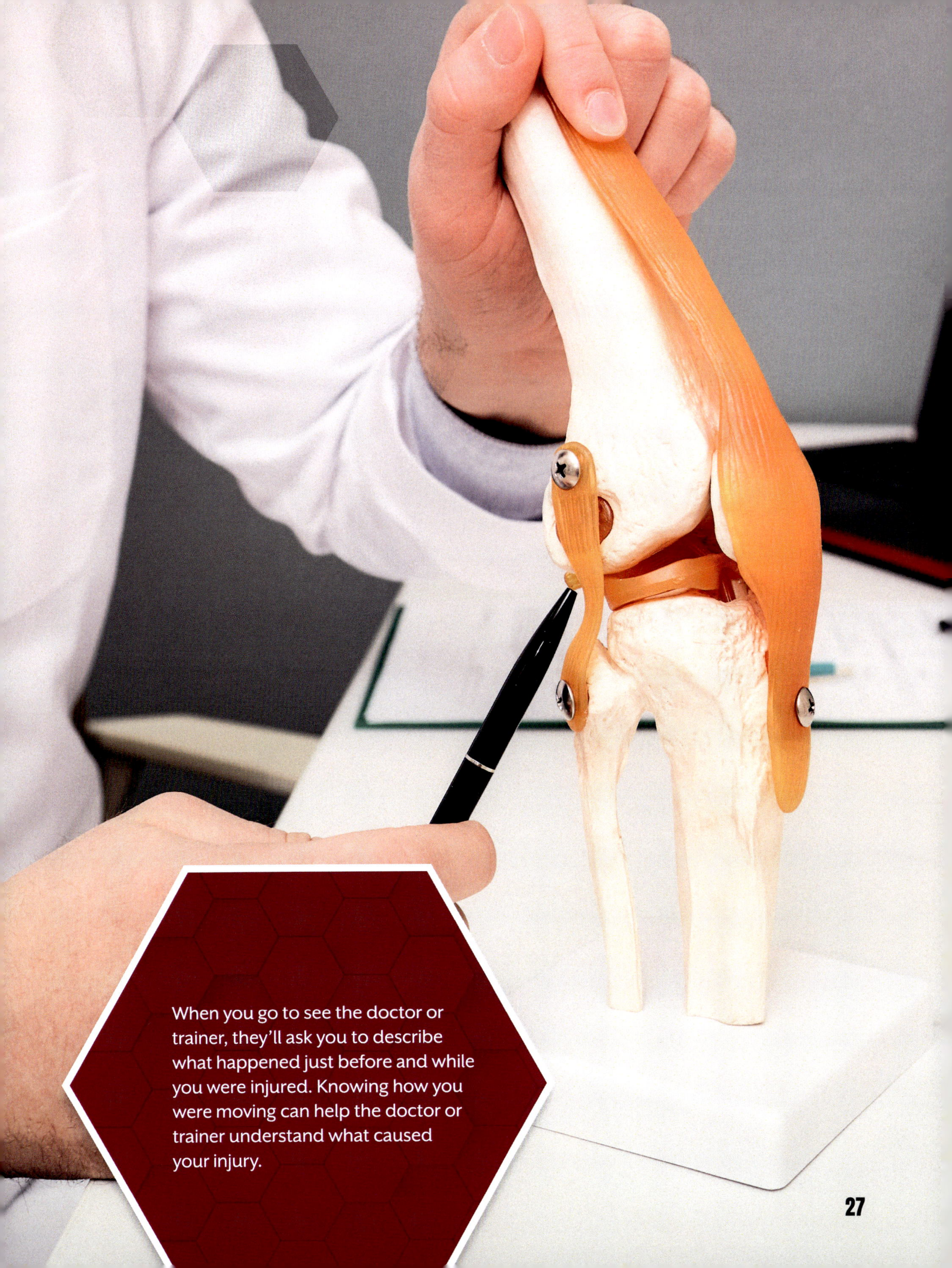

When you go to see the doctor or trainer, they'll ask you to describe what happened just before and while you were injured. Knowing how you were moving can help the doctor or trainer understand what caused your injury.

The doctor or trainer will ask you to stand and walk. You might not be able to do either, and knowing this will also help the doctor diagnose the injury.

The medical professional will also move your leg. One way to test for a Grade 3 ACL tear is to see if your leg can be extended all the way out. With a Grade 3 injury, your ACL has been torn into two pieces, and these pieces get stuck between the femur and tibia. This means that you won't be able to straighten your leg.

The **Lachman test** is another way to check for an ACL tear. During this part of the exam, the medical professional will try to move your tibia forward while holding your femur in place. A healthy ACL stops the tibia from moving too far forward. If your ACL has been completely torn, your tibia will keep moving past where it should stop.

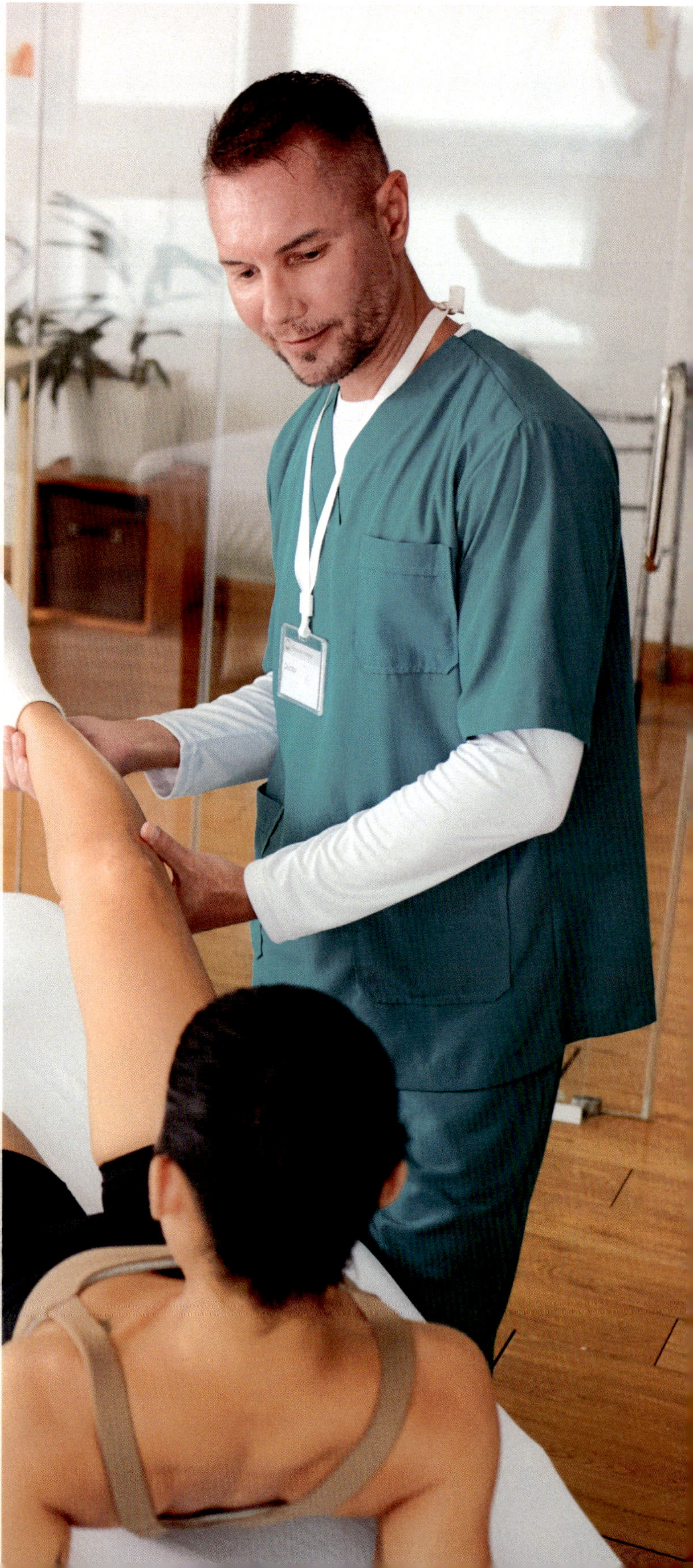

Imaging

There are many ways of seeing inside your body, and doctors may order several tests to help determine how badly your ACL has been torn.

Magnetic Resonance Imaging, commonly called MRI, looks at the muscle and soft tissue. An MRI uses radio waves produced by a computer and a strong magnetic field to create images of the inside of your body. This can help doctors find out how badly the ACL is torn.

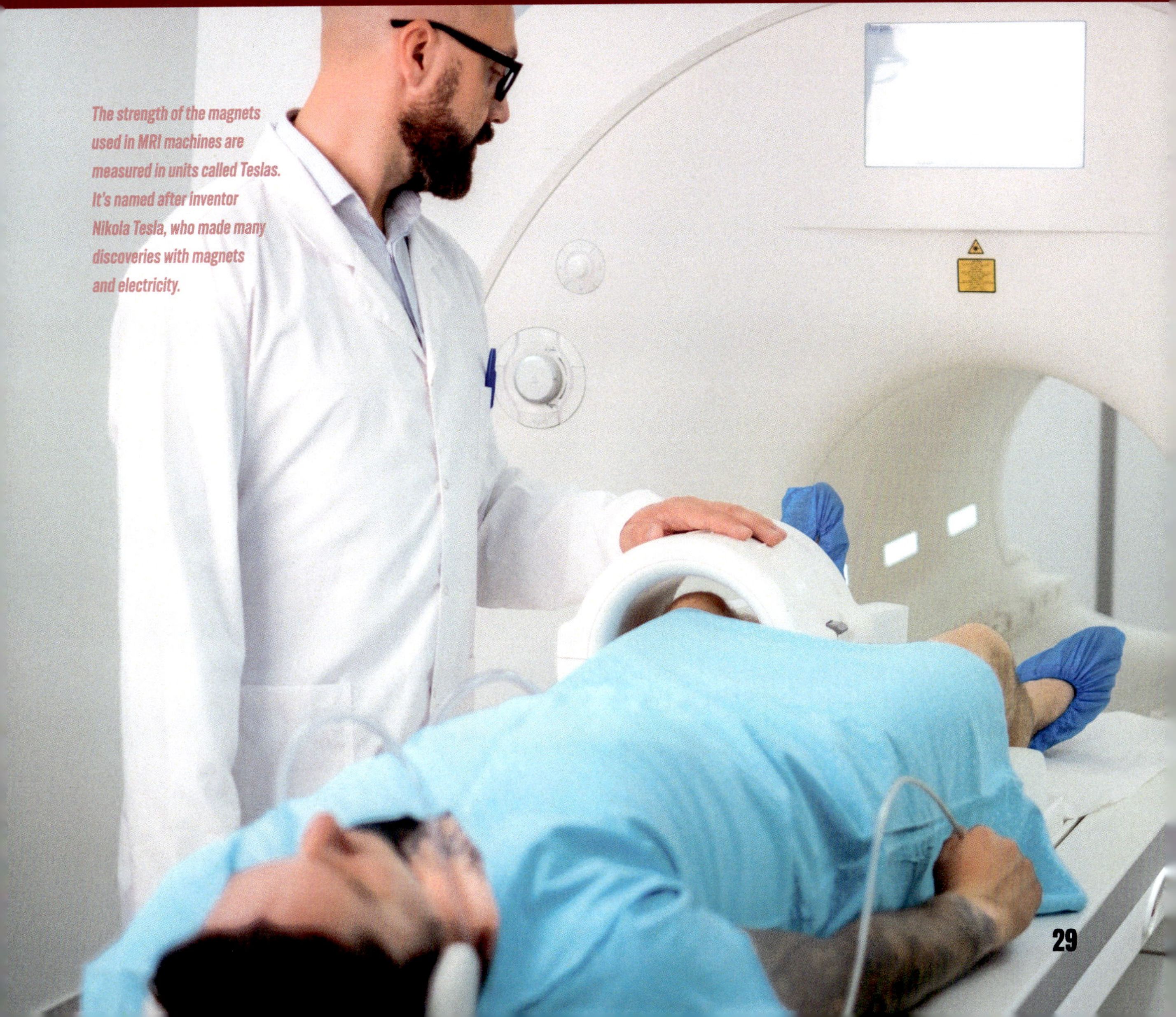

The strength of the magnets used in MRI machines are measured in units called Teslas. It's named after inventor Nikola Tesla, who made many discoveries with magnets and electricity.

Ultrasound is another test that doctors use to check on an injury. Ultrasound, which is also called sonography, uses high frequency sound waves to make an image of the muscle. One benefit to ultrasound is that it can be done while your leg is moving. This can help medical professionals to understand what your muscle looks like in **dynamic** conditions.

If doctors think an avulsion injury may have occurred, they can order an **X-ray**. X-rays take pictures of bone but don't show any muscle or other soft tissue like tendons. Doctors use these images to see if parts of your bone have been removed during an avulsion injury.

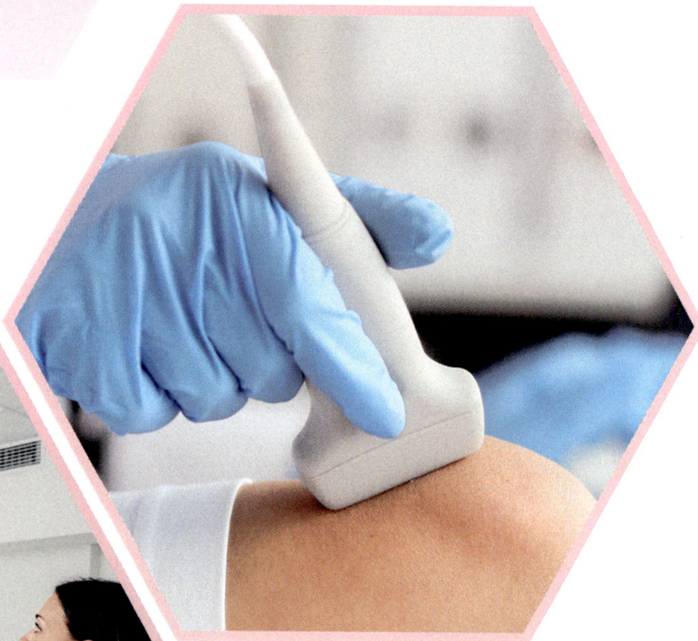

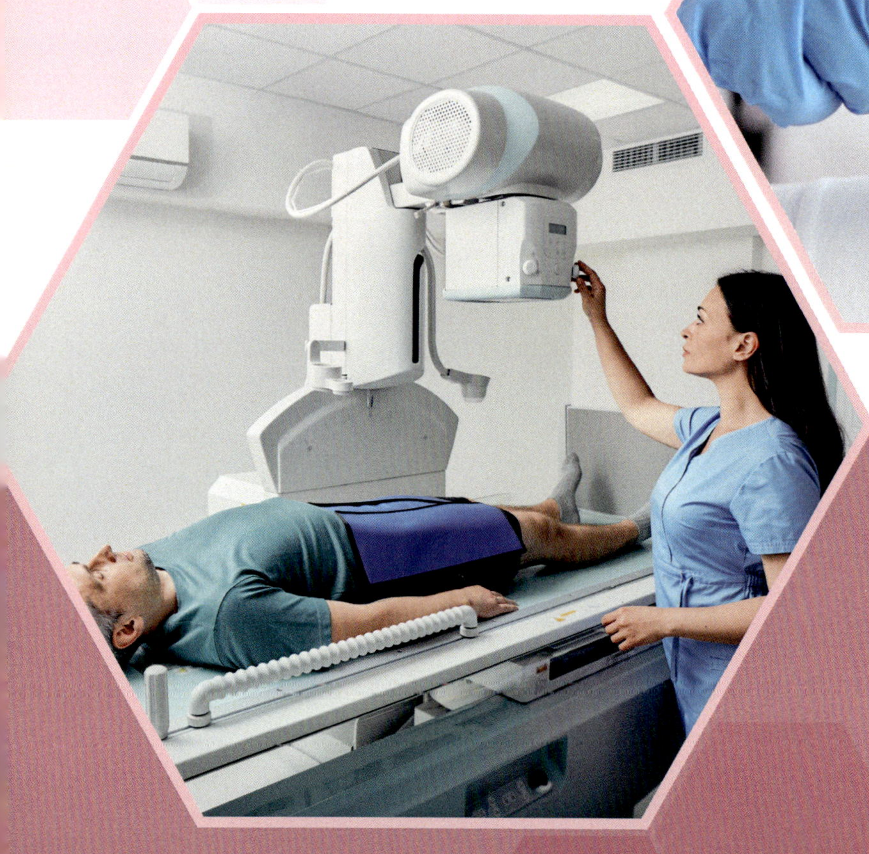

X-rays were discovered by accident. Wilhelm Roentgen, a professor of physics, didn't know what they were, so he named them with an "x" to stand for "unknown."

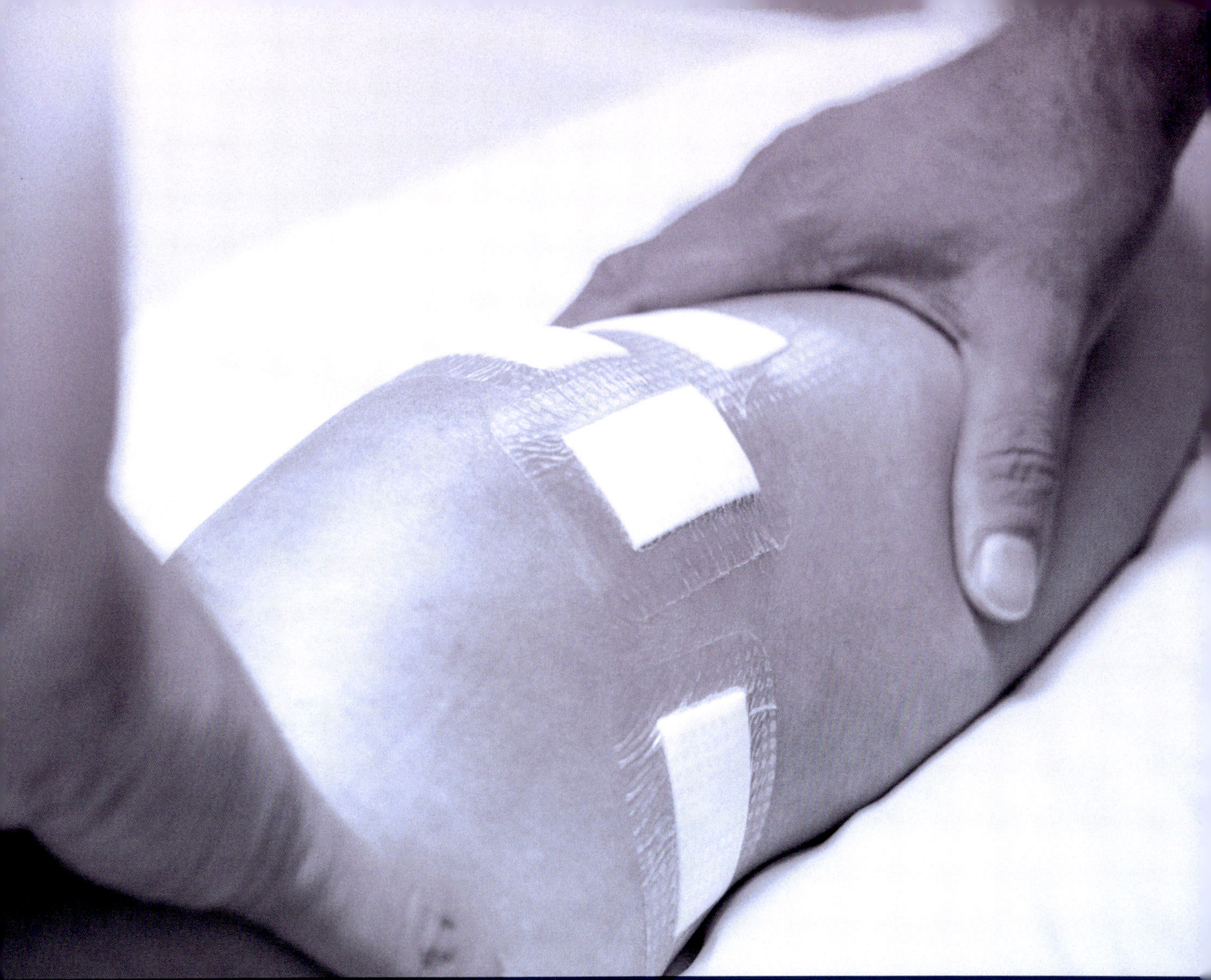

Chapter 6: Treatment

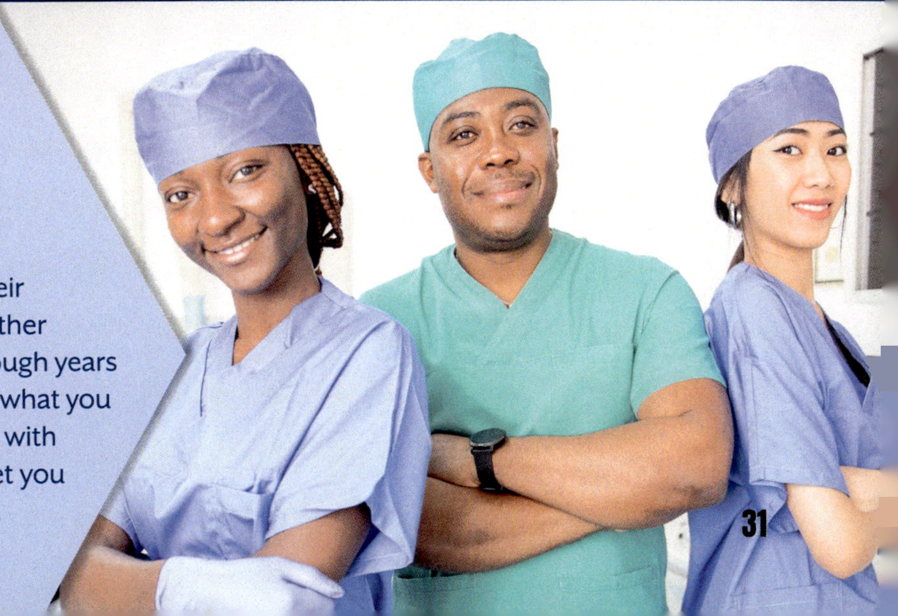

Treatment for an ACL tear depends on how bad the injury is. Mild grade 1 injuries need a different type of treatment plan than a severe Grade 3 injury. You should not try to come up with a treatment plan on their own. Doctors, athletic trainers, and other medical professionals have gone through years of school and training to understand what you need to do to recover. They will work with you to create a customized plan to get you back in the game as soon as possible.

Non-surgical treatment

Grade 1 injuries often heal on their own. The medical professional working with you may tell you to take some time away from your sport and RICE while you're away. RICE stands for

- Rest
- Ice
- Compression
- Elevation

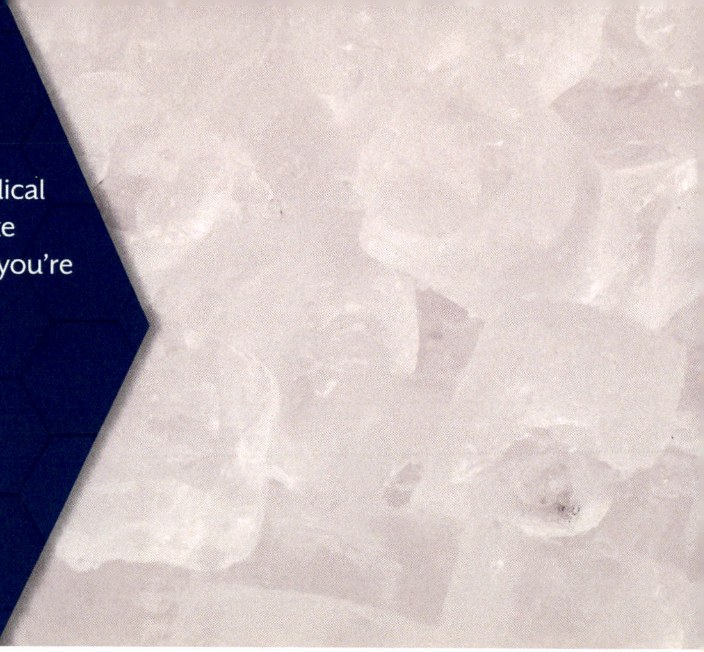

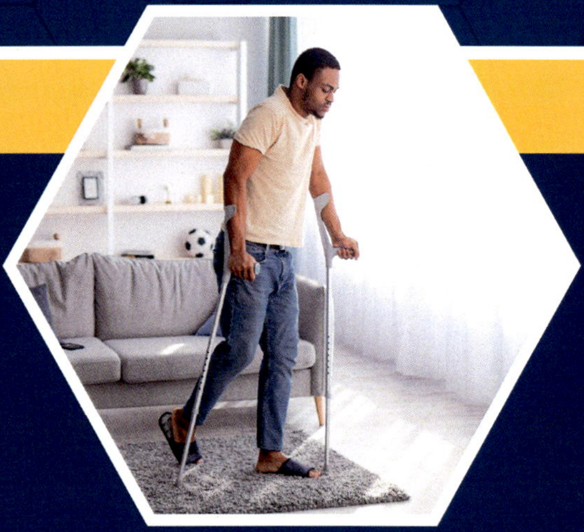

Rest

It is important to stop using your injured leg. You should not try to play sports while hurt.

Ice

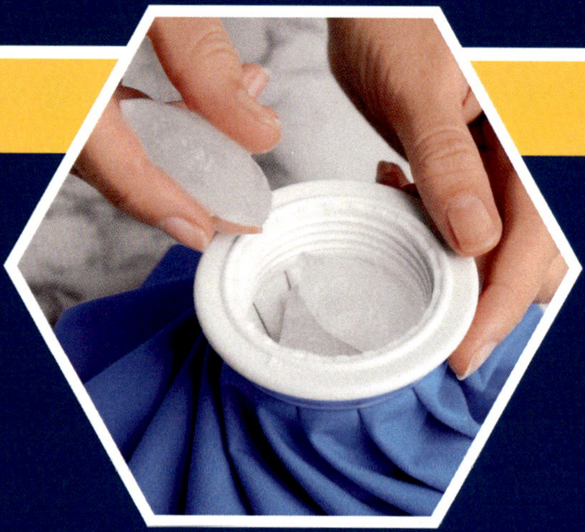

Ice helps keep swelling down and makes the injury hurt less. You should wrap ice packs in a cloth, rather than applying ice directly to your skin. After applying the ice for 20 minutes, wait at least 20 minutes before applying ice again.

If your doctor tells you to ice an injury, they will also tell you how many times to apply the ice. Be sure to listen to your doctor's instructions so that you don't make the injury worse.

RICE was first suggested as a treatment for injuries in 1978. Doctor Gabe Mirkin wrote about each step of in *The Sports Medicine Book*, which was published that year.

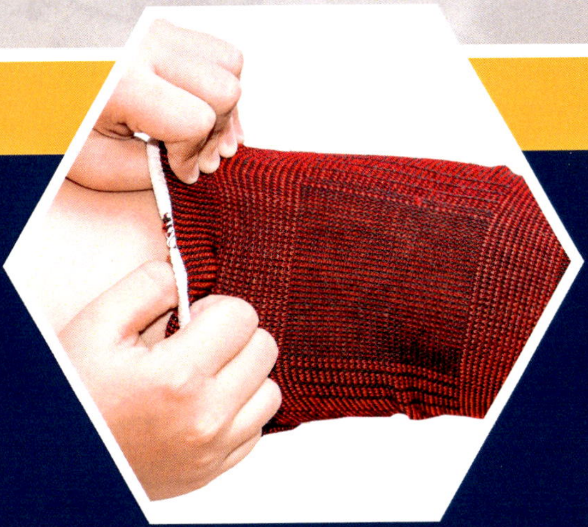

Compression

You may be given instructions to compress your injured knee. Compression helps to decrease swelling. Your doctor or trainer may show you how to wrap your knee with an elastic bandage.

Elevation

Elevating your injured limb means raising it higher than your heart. For an ACL injury, this means that you should be lying down or sitting in order to raise your injured leg. Elevating the injury also helps to decrease swelling.

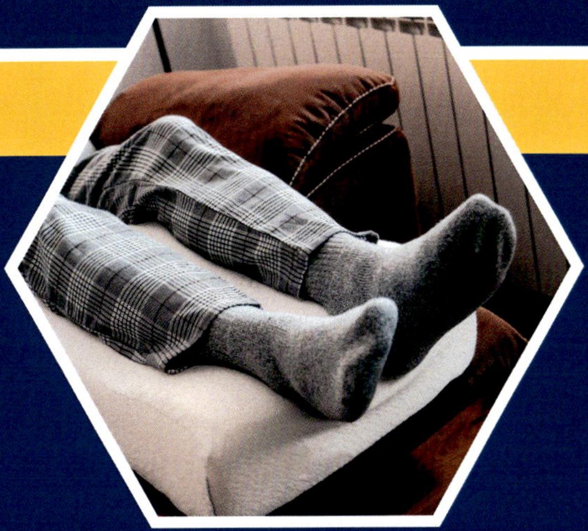

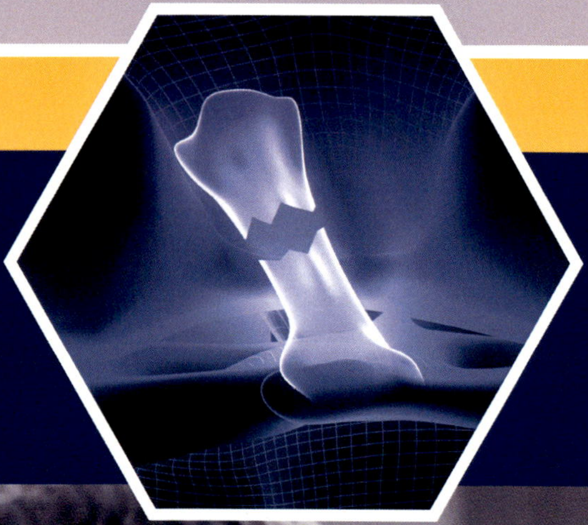

Surgery

Unfortunately, many ACL injuries require surgery. If your ligament is torn, then surgery is needed to replace the ligament. ACL injuries that require surgery usually have a longer recovery time than injuries that can be treated with RICE.

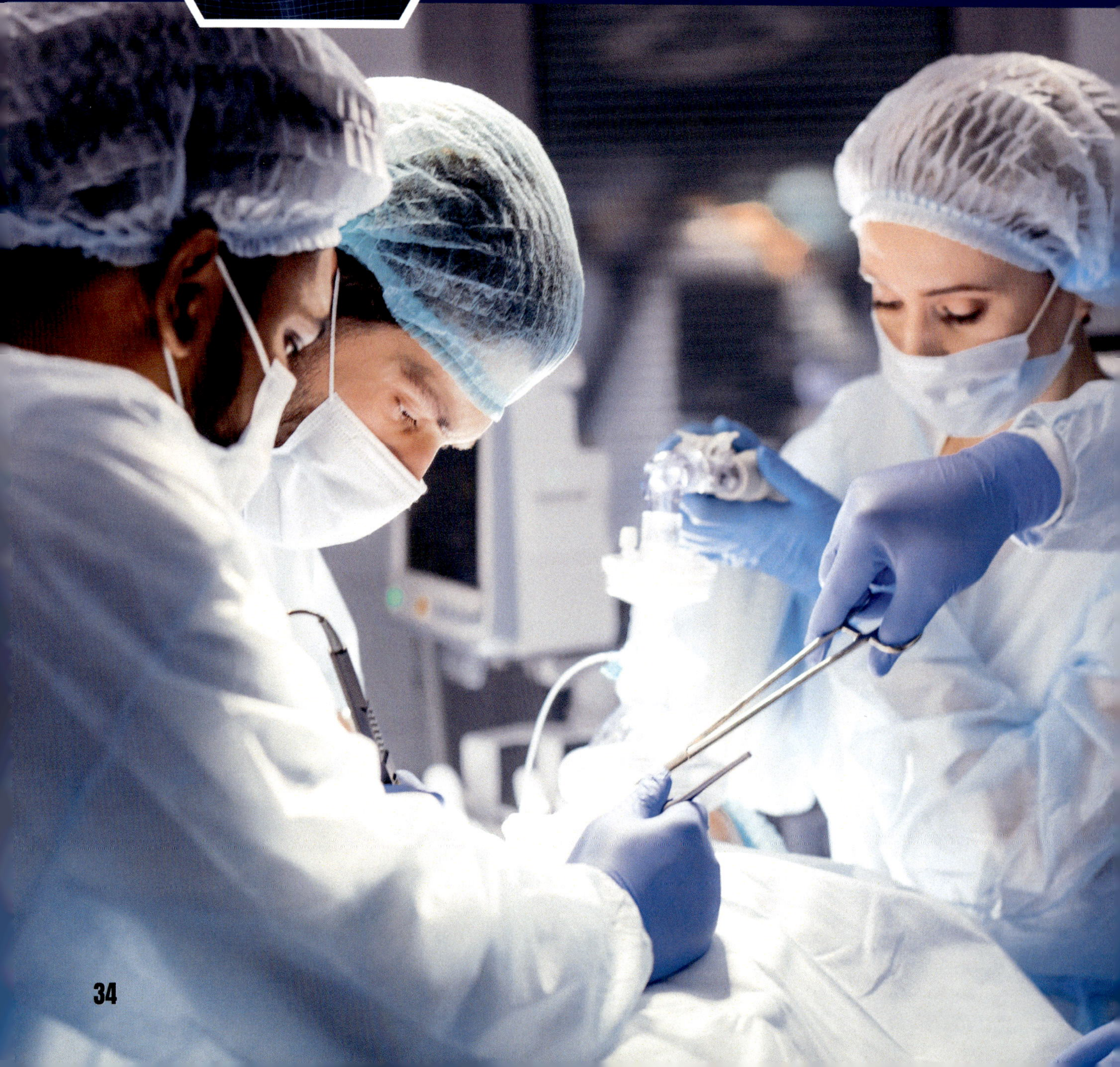

During surgery, a new tendon will be put in place of your old, torn one. Surgeons will remove the injured tendon, drill holes into your bone, and **anchor** a new tendon in place. There are two options for the types of tendons to be used: **allograft** or **autograft**.

Allograft is a donated ligament. This means that it has come from someone else's body instead of yours. Surgeries that use an allograft ligament have faster recovery times, but these ligaments are more likely to be injured later on. Allograft surgeries are generally recommended for older people or athletes who are not as competitive.

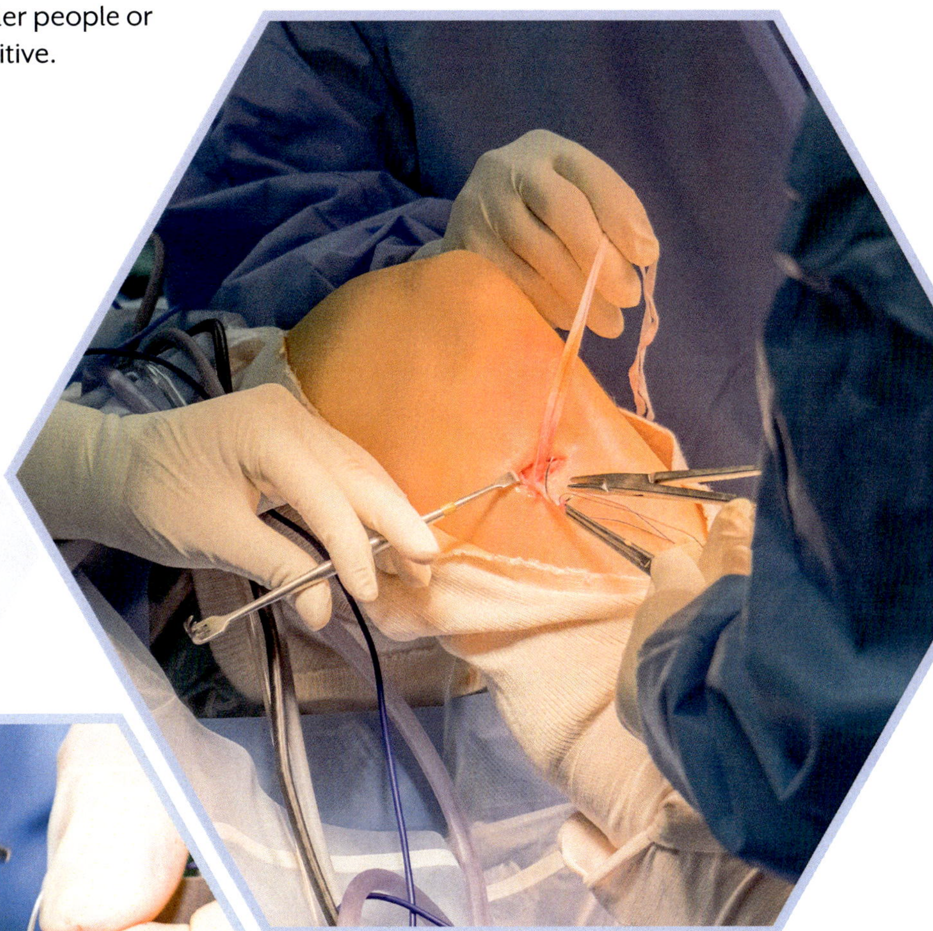

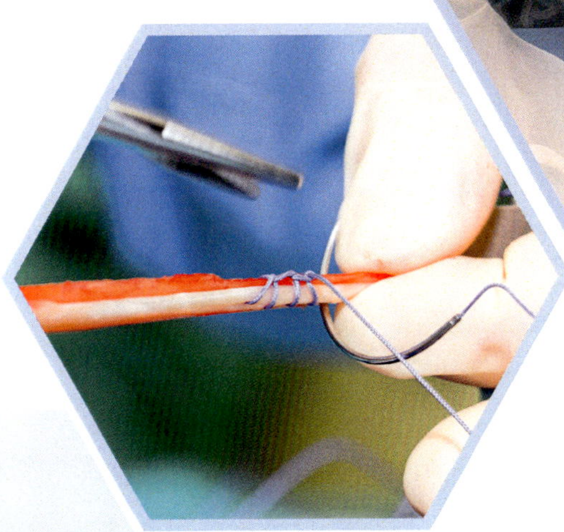

Autograft is a ligament that comes from your own body. A surgeon will take a piece of tissue from your hamstring muscles or other places in your knee. They'll make a new ACL using these pieces of tissue. Because this tissue is coming from your own body, this new ACL is less likely to tear. However, this type of surgery has a longer recovery time than a surgery with an allograft ligament.

Whether surgery or RICE is recommended, it is important that you follow all of the instructions from your doctor or surgeon. Each step of the treatment process is important and is designed to help you recover completely. The doctors and surgeons want to see you return to sports quickly, and following the treatment plan is the fastest way there.

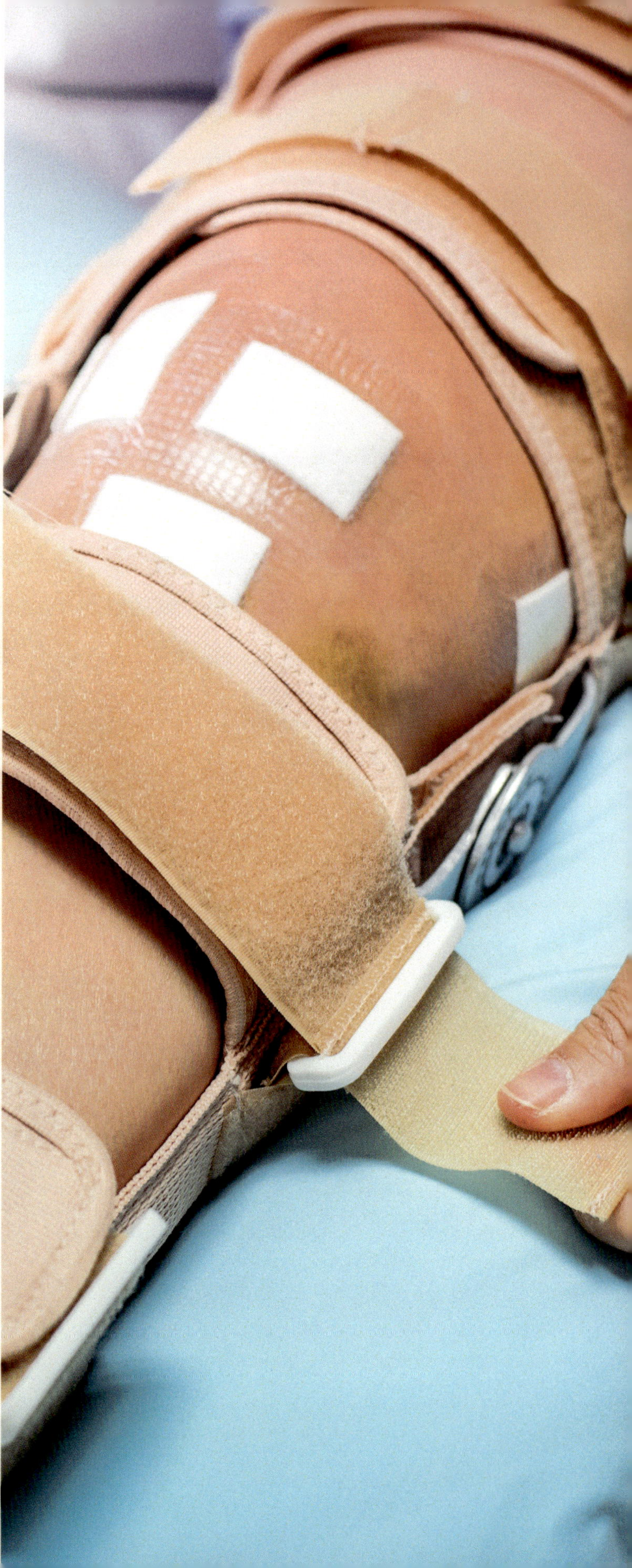

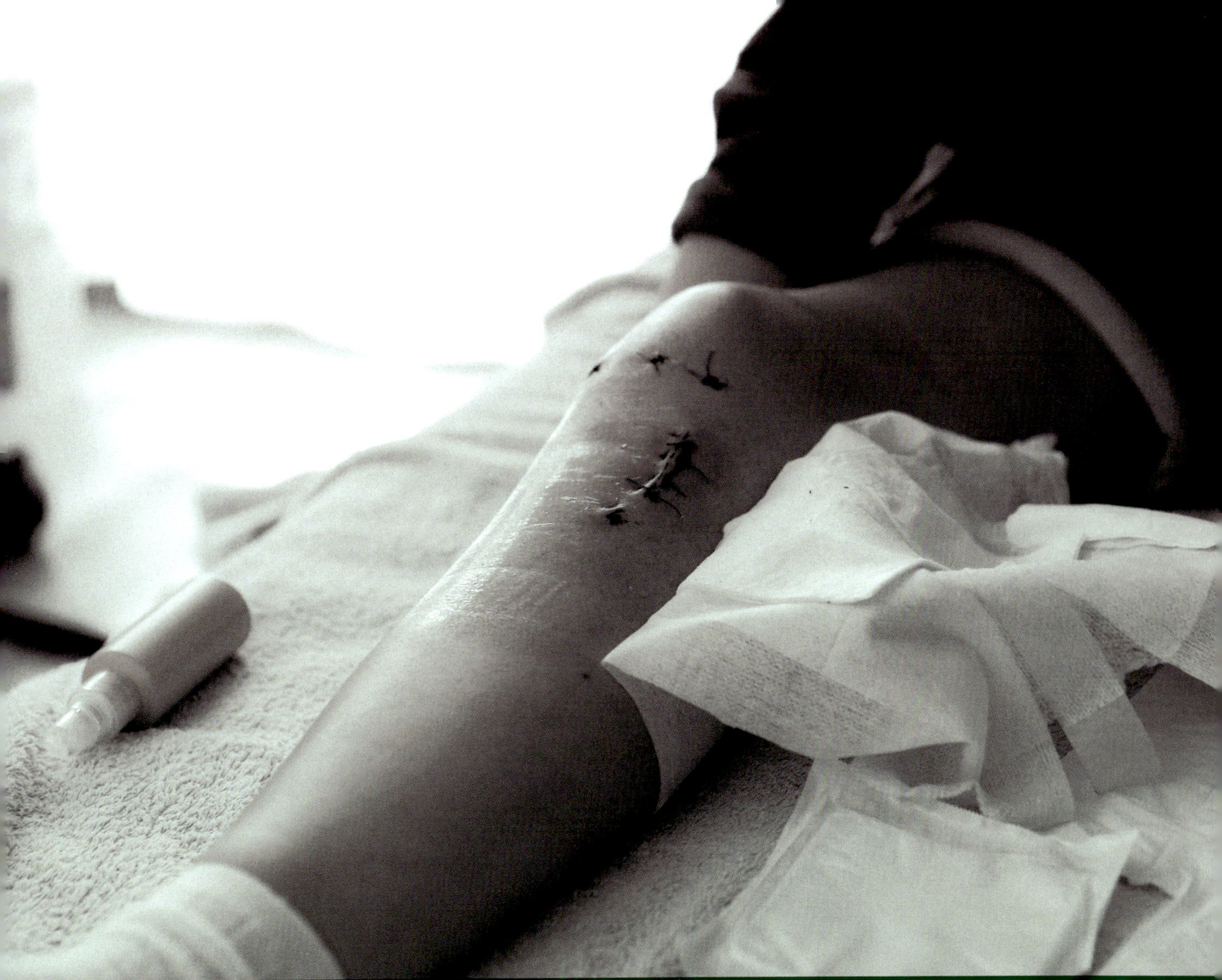

Chapter 7: Recovery

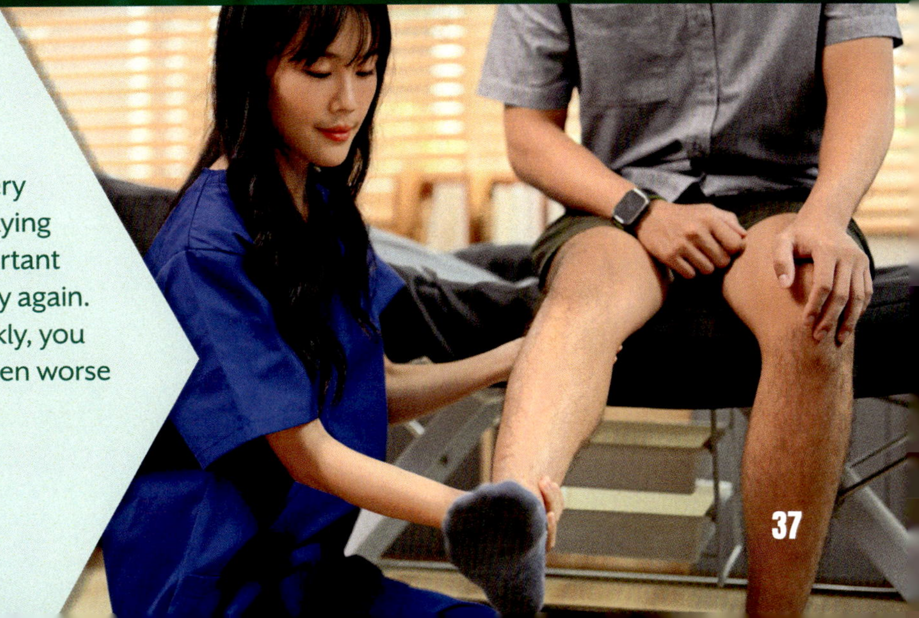

ACL injuries can have a long recovery time. It can be hard to sit out of playing sports while you heal, but it's important to fully recover before trying to play again. If you rush back to sports too quickly, you could reinjure yourself, possibly even worse than before.

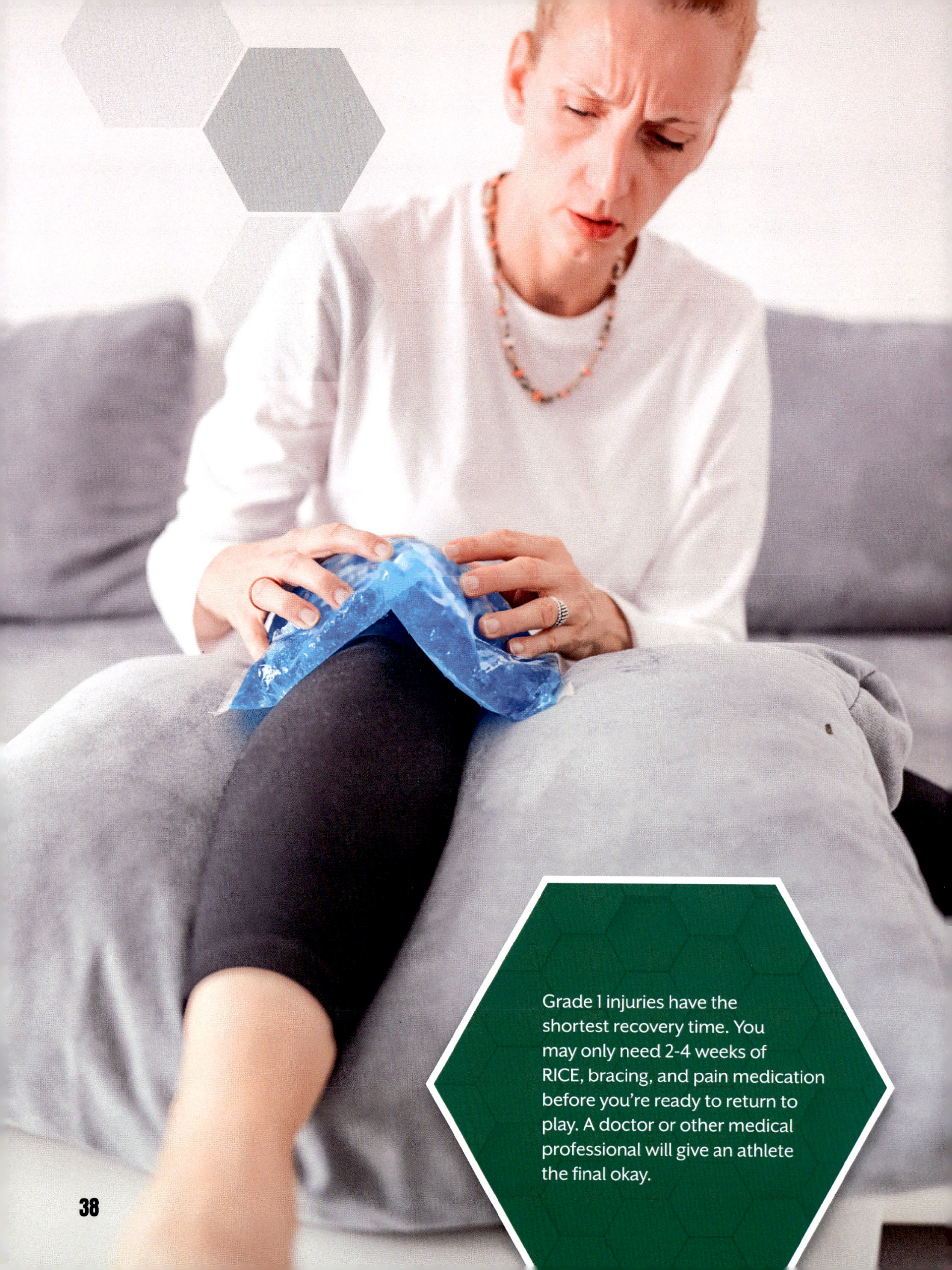

Grade 1 injuries have the shortest recovery time. You may only need 2-4 weeks of RICE, bracing, and pain medication before you're ready to return to play. A doctor or other medical professional will give an athlete the final okay.

ACL injuries that require surgery will have longer recovery times. First your wound needs to heal, and then you must build back muscle tone and flexibility. Working with a physical therapist is an important part of recovery for a severe ACL injury. During **physical therapy,** you'll stretch your leg and work the ligaments and muscles of your knee. Exercises help your leg grow strong again. Stretches work to increase your knee's **range of motion.** Other exercises will help you regain balance and stability.

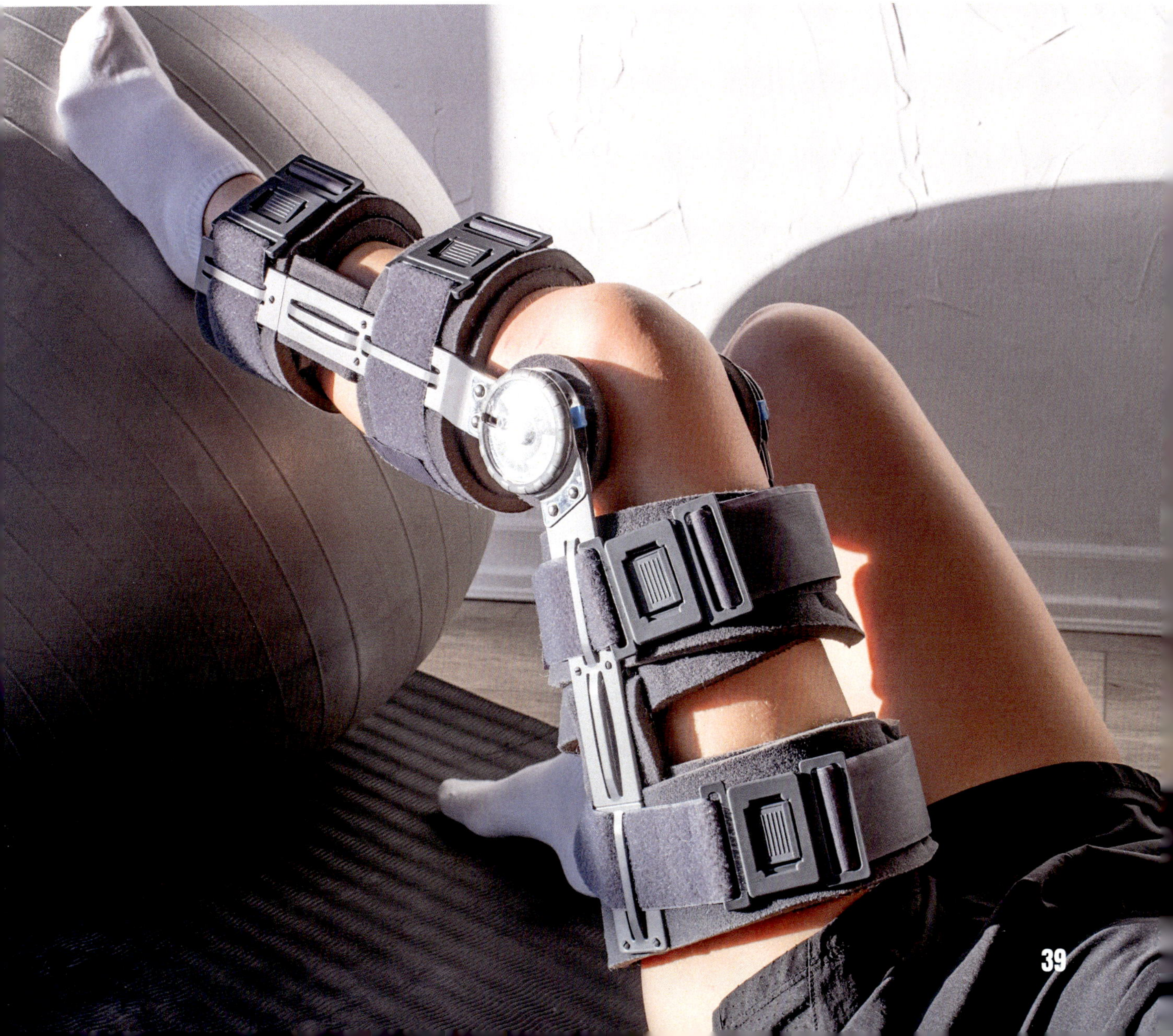

Recovery for Women and Girls

Female athletes may have additional goals while recovering from ACL injuries. Physical therapists or athletic trainers may recommend exercises to change how you land after a jump or how to change direction suddenly. They may also suggest exercises for your ankle and hip. Strengthening both of these areas will help keep your knee stable and supported.

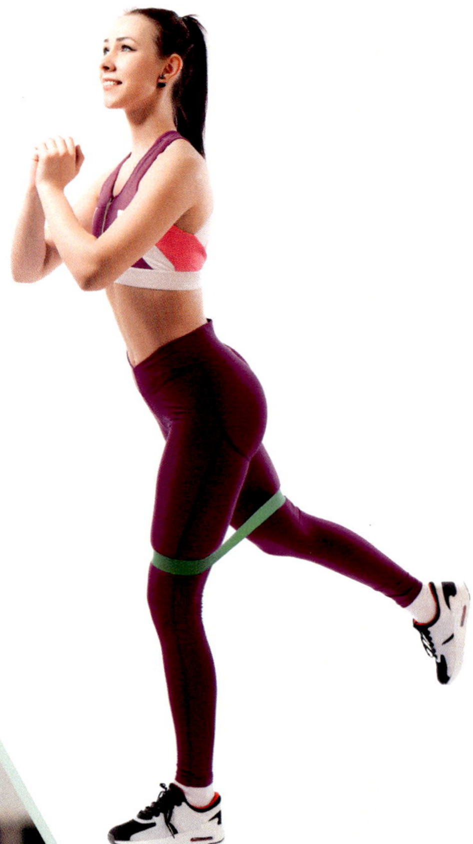

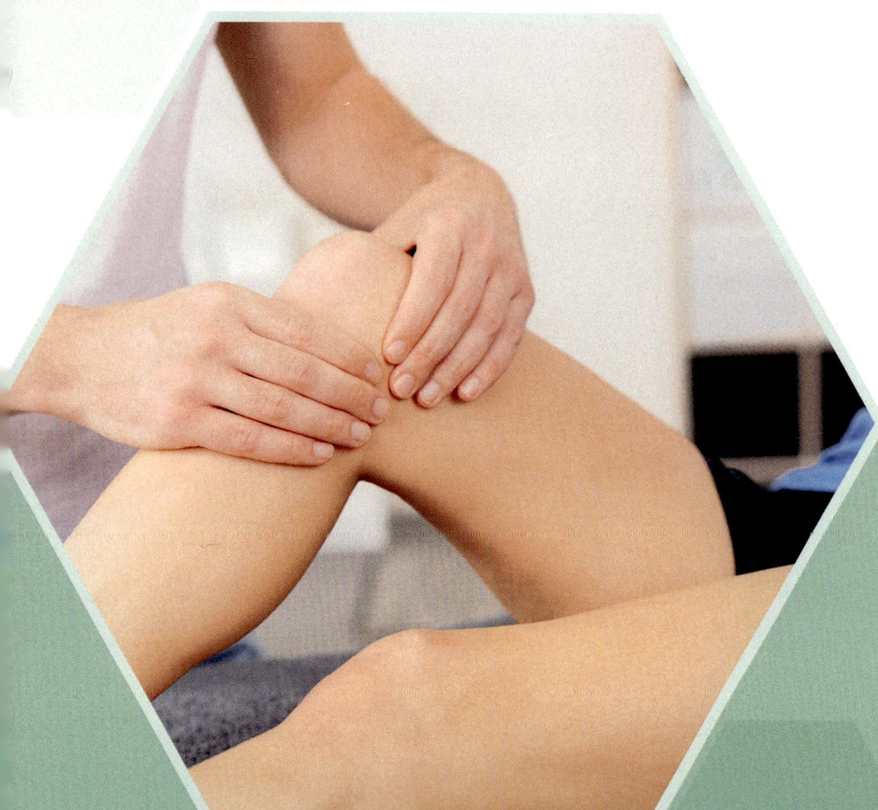

One exercise a physical therapist may suggest is called a heel slide.

1.) *Sit on the floor with your legs stretched out in front of you*

2.) *Bend one knee while sliding your heel across the floor*

3.) *Slide your heel along the floor back to the starting position*

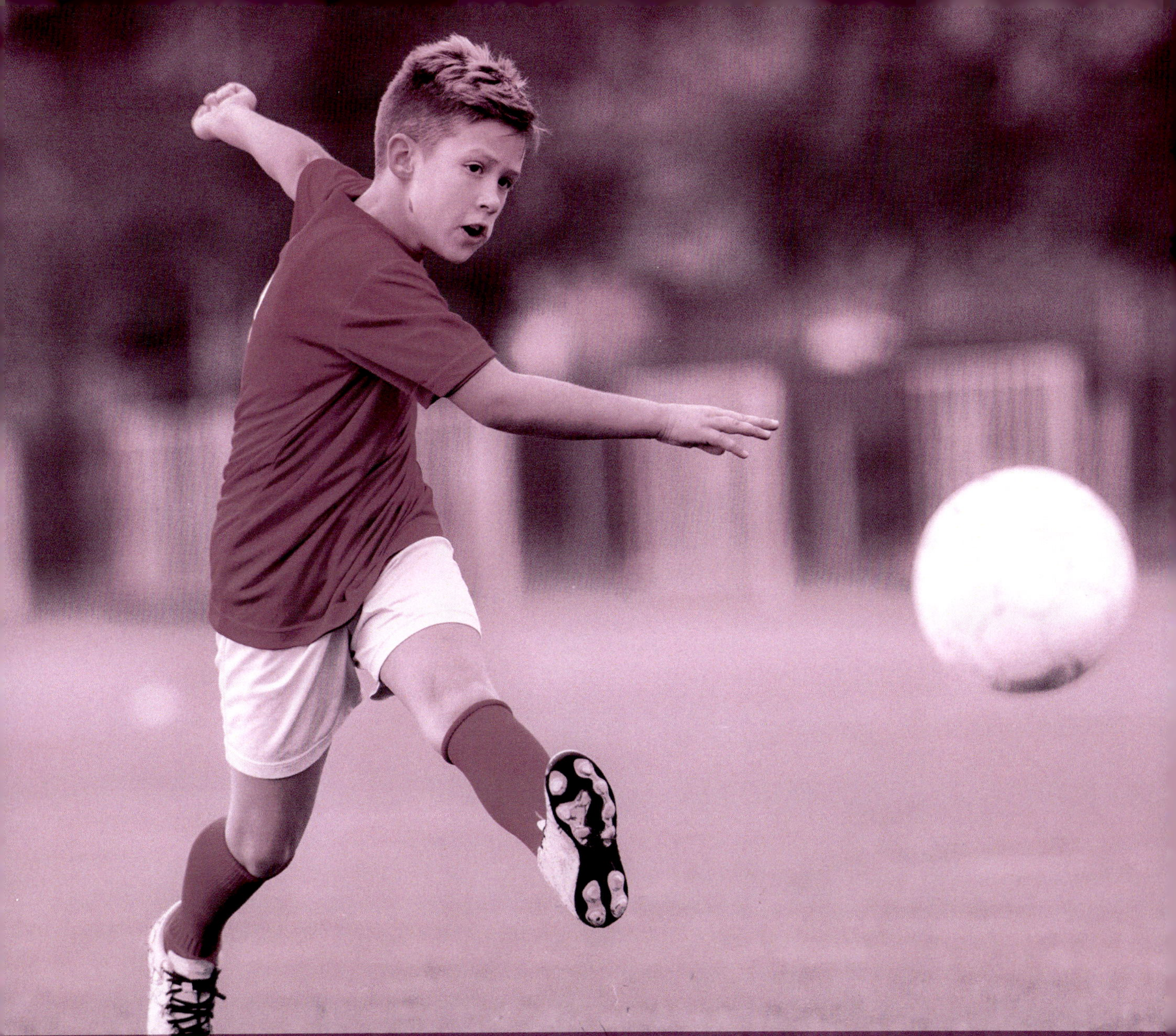

Chapter 8: Prevention

ACL injures happen suddenly, but there are several ways to prevent these injuries. Always make sure that your gear fits correctly. Playing in shoes that are too tight or too loose can change the way you jump, land, pivot, and run. You want to make sure that your body can move properly. Have someone experienced in athletic gear help fit you for the correct sizes.

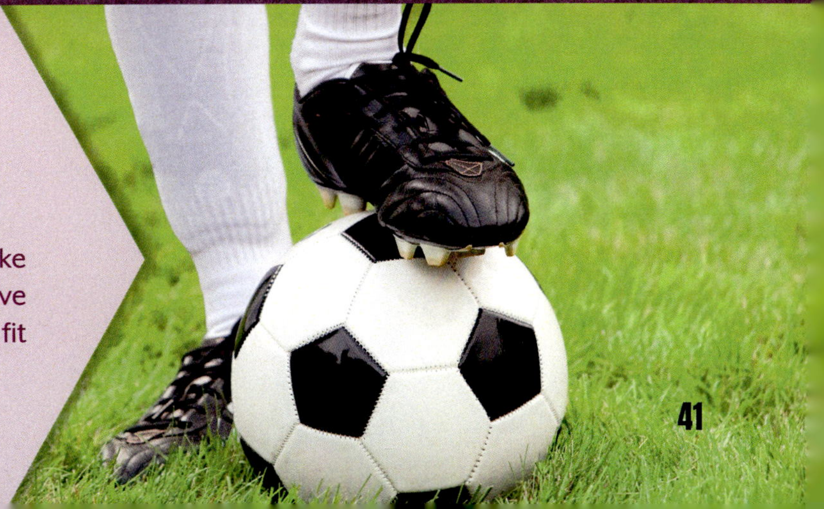

Take the time to stretch, warm up, and cool down. Ligaments, muscles, and tendons that are used too quickly are more likely to be injured. It's important to make sure that the muscles which surround and support your knee joint are healthy and strong.

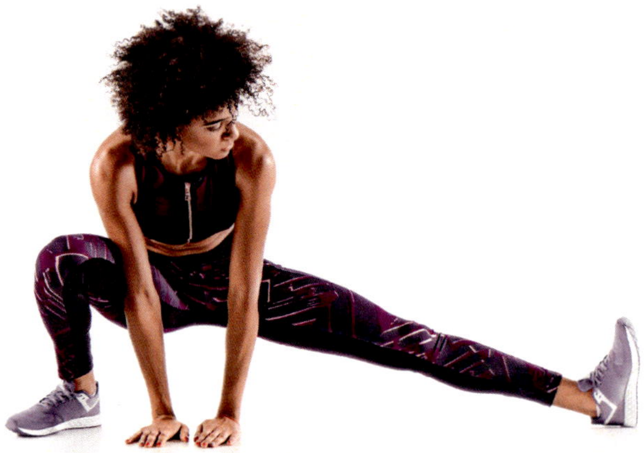

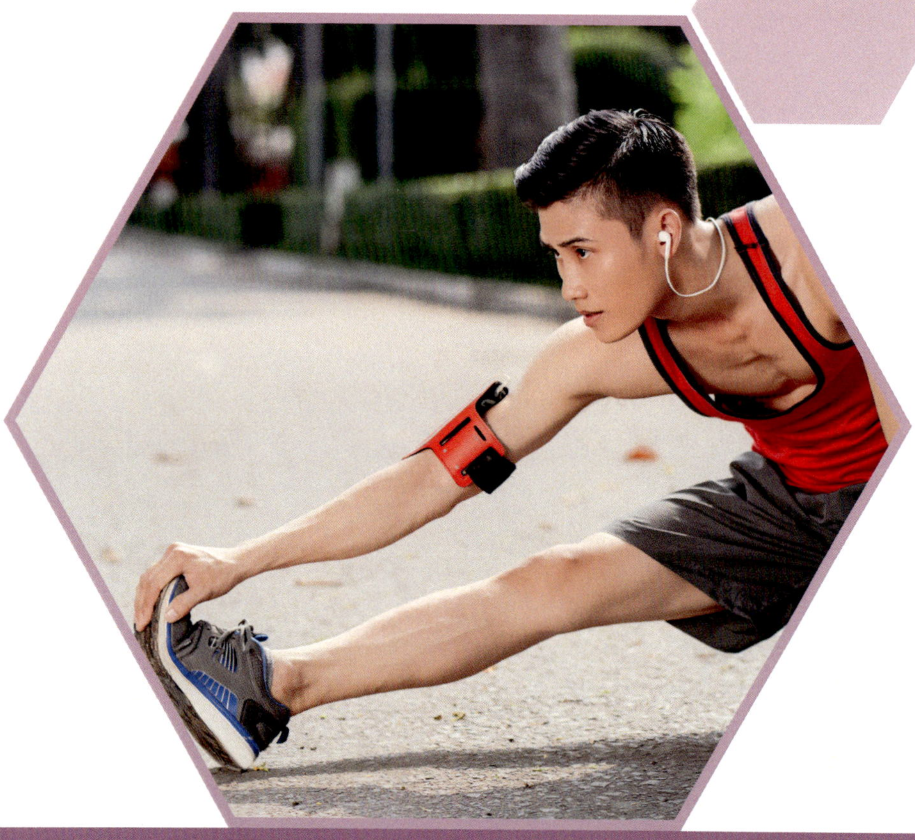

ACL injuries and tears are common sports injuries. Any athlete who runs, jumps, or makes sudden changes in direction is at risk. Contact sports like football, basketball, and soccer also increase the risk of this injury. But understanding how your body works and making sure to stretch and exercise weak areas will help prevent this injury.

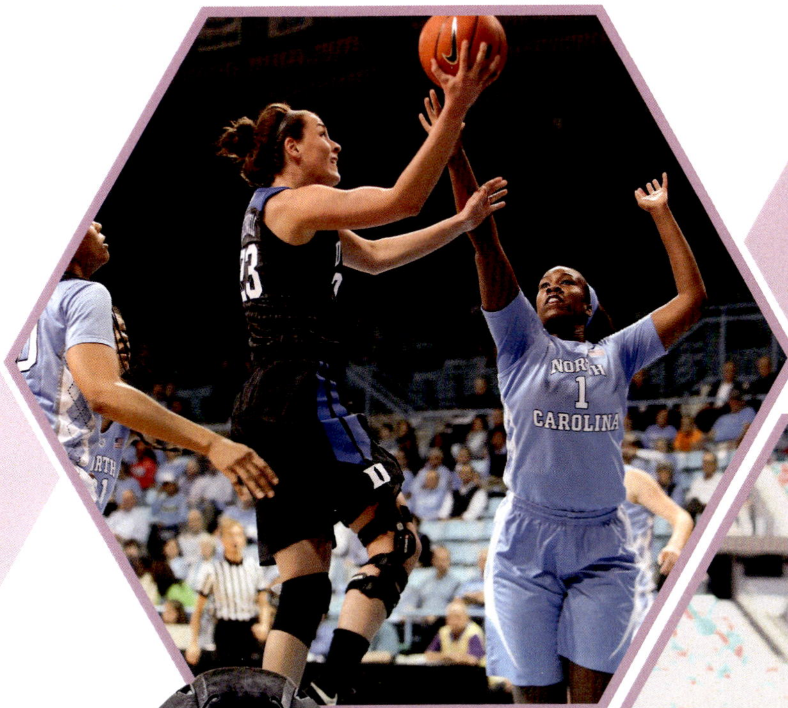

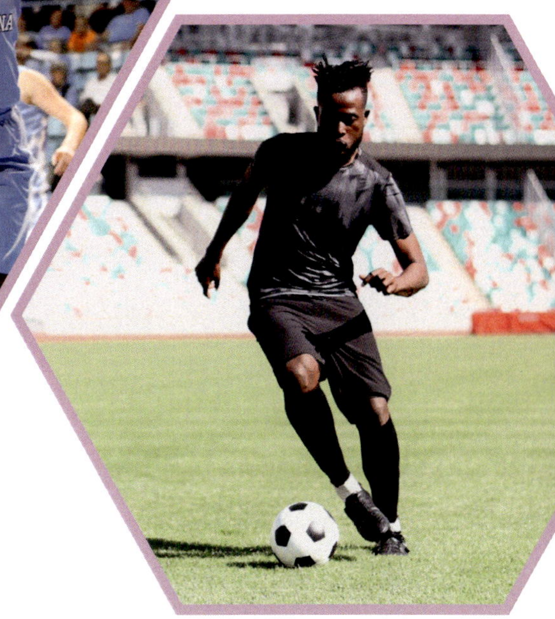

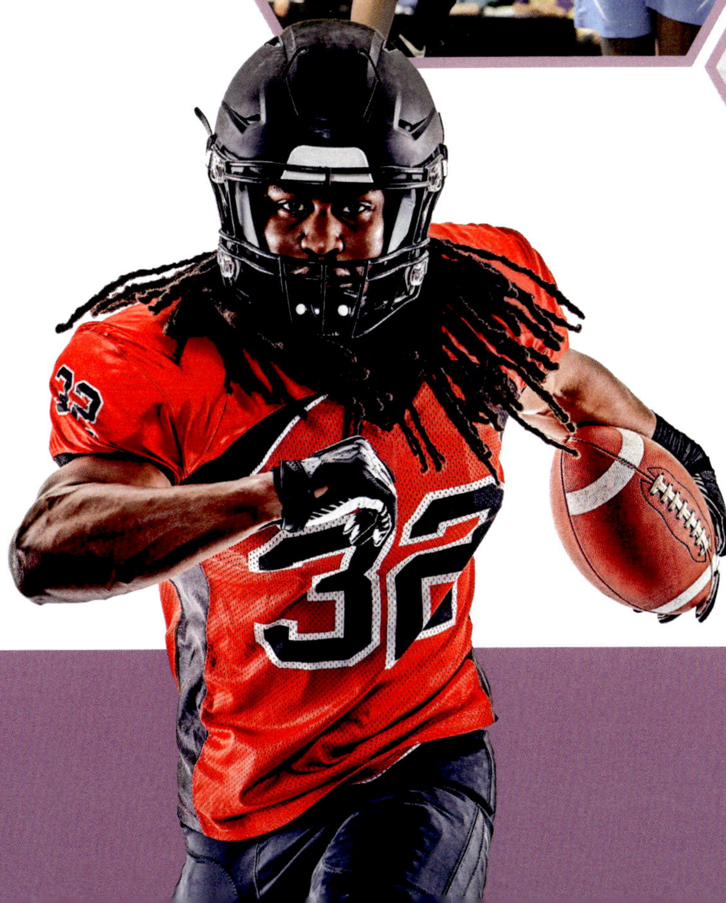

Glossary

allograft (AL-uh-graft): Tissue taken from one person and used to heal another person

anatomy (un-NAT-uh-mee): The study of the parts of the human body

anterior (an-TEER-ee-er): In front of

autograft (AW-tuh-graft): Tissue taken from one part of the body and used to heal a different part of the same person

avulsion injury (uh-VUHL-shun IN-juh-ree): An injury where part of the bone is torn away

anchor (ANG-ker): A device for holding something in place

dynamic (dhay-NAM-ik): In motion

extend (ik-STEND): To make the full length

femur (FEE-mur): The upper leg bone and the longest bone in the human body

flex (fleks): To bend

hormones (HAWR-mohnz): Chemicals produced by the human body to act as signals to other parts of the body

hypothesis (hahy-POTH-uh-sis): A guess based on some reasoning or prior thought

joint (joint): Where two or more bones meet

lachman test (LAHK-man test): A way to evaluate if the ACL is injured by pulling the tibia forward compared to the femur

ligament (LIG-uh-muhnts): Soft structures which connect bones with other bones

magnetic resonance imaging (mag-NET-ik REZ-uh-nuhns IM-uh-jing): A machine that uses magnets to take images of the soft parts inside the human body, commonly known as MRI

mobile joint (MOH-buhl joints): A joint whose purpose is to move

muscle (MUH-sels): Soft tissue in the human body which contracts to move bones

pelvis (PEL-vis): A group of bones that make up the lower torso, commonly known as the hip bones

physical therapy (FIZ-i-kuhl THER-uh-pee): A branch of medicine that helps patients regain and main health through exercises and stretches

range of motion (reynj uhv MOH-shun): How far a joint is able to move

screw home mechanism (skroo hohm MEK-uh-niz-uhm): The rotation of the femur on the tibia to stabilize the knee joint

tibia (TIB-ee-uh): The long bone of the lower leg. This is commonly called the shin bone

ultrasound (UHL-truh-sound): High frequency sound waves that are used to see inside the human body

X-ray (EKS-rey): Electromagnetic radiation with a shorter wavelength than light that can show images of hard tissue like bone

Index

Comprehension Questions

1. What does "cruciate" mean?
    a. To cut
    b. To cross
    c. To chop
2. True or false: ACL tears are common sports injuries.
3. The knee joint is
    a. A hinge joint
    b. A ball and socket joint
    c. A saddle joint
4. True or false: An athlete will be able to walk with a Grade 3 ACL tear
5. True or false: Grade 3 hamstring injuries are the most severe.
6. RICE stands for
    a. Running, Ice skating, Climbing, and Equestrian.
    b. Red, Inflamed, Contusion, and Enlarged.
    c. Rest, Ice, Compression, and Elevation.
7. One way to prevent ACL injuries is to
    a. Eat raisins
    b. Increase muscle strength
    c. Exercise in shorts
8. True or false: contact sports increase the risk of ACL tears

1. b 2. true 3. a 4. false 5. true 6. c 7. b 8. true

About the Author

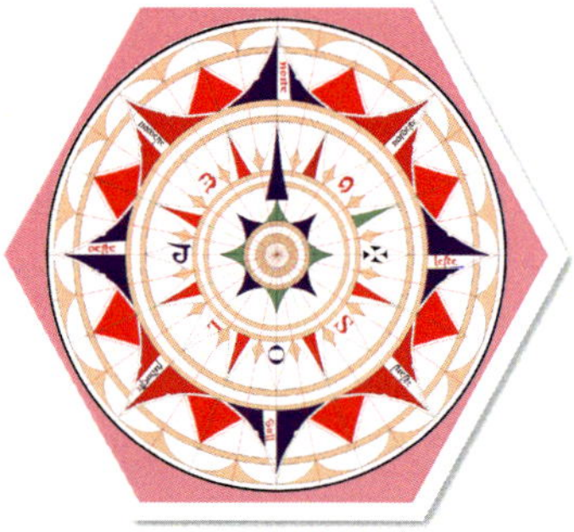

India James writes about science, technology, and math for young readers. She loves when science comes together with sports. India lives in Ohio with her family.

Author: India James

Editor: Ellen Rodger

Design: Jen Bowers

IMAGE CREDITS

Shutterstock: Cover and title page ©2013 CLIPAREA l Custom media (p.4, p.11, p.34), ©2024 Pro.Sto (p.43), ©2016 Kaspars Grinvalds (p.5), ©2023 MillaF (p.20); p.4 ©2018 Pressmaster; p.5 ©2024 Atiketta Sangasaeng; p.6 ©2022 PeopleImages.com-Yuri A, ©2007 Dennis Ku; p.7 ©Viktoriia_P, ©2018 Dmytro Zinkevych; p.8 ©2019 Orla; p.9 ©2022 PeopleImages.com-Yuri A, ©2016 Africa Studio; p.10 ©2023 BigBlueStudio, ©2016 Dmytro Vietrov; p.11 ©2024 Axel_Kock; p.12 ©2016 Cast Of Thousands, ©2019 Regreto; p.13 ©2024 TippaPatt, ©2020 Margaret Kite; p.14 ©2016 Debby Wong; p.15 ©2024 Ringo Chiu; p.16 ©2018 marino bocelli; p.17 ©Double Brain; p.18 ©2024 Anton Vierietin; p.19 ©2024 muse studio; p.20 ©2018 Landscapes From The Sky; p.21 ©2022 MDV Edwards, ©Pepermpron (p.22, 23); p.22 ©2017 Piyada Jaiaree, ©2019 Lumena (p.23); p.23 ©2020 November27; p.24 ©2020 Roman Chazov; p.25 ©2021 Steve Jacobson, ©2015 Andrey_Popov; p.26 ©2021 Ground Picture, ©2024 Daniel Hoz; p.27 ©2021 Peakstock; p.28 ©2023 Dragon Images; p.29 ©2021 fizkes, ©2019 Nejron Photo; p.30 ©2023 H_Ko, ©2022 Peakstock; p.31 ©2019 November27, ©2022 Media Lens King; p.32 ©2020 Wira SHK, ©2021 Prostock-studio, ©2019 New Africa; p.33 ©2014 Tewan Banditrakkanka, ©2023 nito; p.34 ©2018 UfaBizPhoto; p.35 ©2016 Samrith Na Lumpoon, ©2016 Raul Topan; p.36 ©2019 November27; p.37 ©2022 Mihai Blanaru, ©2024 Prathankarnpap; p.38 ©2019 AstroStar; p.39 ©2022 ilona.shorokhova; p.40 ©2019 Everyonephoto Studio, ©2015 stockfour; p.41 ©2016 Fotokostic, ©2009 Le Do; p.42 ©2017 RomarioIen, ©2016 Dragon Images; p.43 ©2016 Debby Wong, © 2018 OSTILL is Franck Camhi; p.48 About the Author image ©Alvesgaspar

Crabtree Publishing

crabtreebooks.com 800-387-7650

In Canada: We acknowledge the financial support of the Government of Canada through the Canada Book Fund for our publishing activities.

Hardcover 978-1-0398-8079-5
Paperback 978-1-0398-8440-3
Ebook (pdf) 978-1-0398-8199-0
Epub 978-1-0398-8319-2

Published in Canada
Crabtree Publishing
616 Welland Avenue
St. Catharines, Ontario
L2M 5V6

Published in the United States
Crabtree Publishing
347 Fifth Avenue
Suite 1402-145
New York, New York, 10016

Library and Archives Canada Cataloguing in Publication
Available at Library and Archives Canada

Library of Congress Cataloging-in-Publication Data
Available at the Library of Congress

Printed in the USA/CP2025